Temporomandibular Joint Surgery

Editors
DANIEL P. CARUSO
BRIANA J. BURRIS

ATLAS OF THE ORAL AND MAXILLOFACIAL SURGERY CLINICS OF NORTH AMERICA

www.oralmaxsurgeryatlas.theclinics.com

Consulting Editor
RUI P. FERNANDES

September 2026 • Volume 34 • Number 2

ELSEVIER

1818 Market Street • Suite 3323 • Philadelphia, Pennsylvania, 19103-2899
http://www.theclinics.com

ATLAS OF THE ORAL AND MAXILLOFACIAL SURGERY CLINICS OF NORTH AMERICA Volume 34, Number 2 September 2026 ISSN 1061-3315 ISBN-13: 978-0-443-47470-5

Editor: Patrick Manley; p.manley@elsevier.com
Developmental Editor: Gaurav Singh

Reprints. For copies of 100 or more of articles in this publication, please contact the Commercial Reprints Department, Elsevier Inc., 360 Park Avenue South, New York, NY 10010-1710. Tel.: 212-633-3874; Fax: 212-633-3820; E-mail: reprints@elsevier.com.

Publishing Office: *Atlas of the Oral and Maxillofacial Surgery Clinics of North America* (ISSN 1061-3315) is published biannually by Elsevier Inc., 1818 Market Street, Philadelphia, PA 19103, United States. Months of issue are March and September. Periodicals postage paid at New York, NY and additional mailing offices. Subscription prices are $489.00 for international individual, $408.00 for US individual, $429.00 for Canadian individual; $220.00 for international student, $100.00 for US student and Canadian student. For institutional access pricing please contact Customer Service via the contact information below. Foreign air speed delivery is included in all *Clinics* subscription prices. All prices are subject to change without notice. Orders, claims, and journal inquiries: Please visit our Support Hub page https://service.elsevier.com for assistance.

Atlas of the Oral and Maxillofacial Surgery Clinics of North America is covered in *MEDLINE/PubMed (Index Medicus).*

Contributors

CONSULTING EDITOR

RUI P. FERNANDES, MD, DMD, FACS, FRCS(Ed)
Clinical Professor and Chief, Division of Head and Neck Surgery, Program Director, Head and Neck Oncologic Surgery and Microvascular Reconstruction Fellowship, Departments of Oral and Maxillofacial Surgery, Neurosurgery, and Orthopaedic Surgery and Rehabilitation, University of Florida Health Science Center, University of Florida College of Medicine, Jacksonville, Florida, USA

EDITORS

DANIEL P. CARUSO, MD, DDS
Assistant Professor, Division of Head and Neck Surgery, Department of Oral and Maxillofacial Surgery, University of Florida College of Medicine–Jacksonville, Jacksonville, Florida, USA

BRIANA J. BURRIS, DDS, FACS
Program Director, Oral and Maxillofacial Surgery Residency Training Program, Department of Oral and Maxillofacial Surgery, Massachusetts General Hospital, Instructor, Harvard Medical School and Harvard School of Dental Medicine, Boston, Massachusetts, USA

AUTHORS

JASON ADAM, DDS
Resident, Department of Oral and Maxillofacial Surgery, Massachusetts General Hospital, Harvard School of Dental Medicine, Boston, Massachusetts, USA

DAVID AHN, DMD, FACS
Surgeon, Department of Oral and Maxillofacial Surgery, University of California, San Francisco VA Medical Center, San Francisco, California, USA

MESHAL AL MUNIF, DDS, SBOMFS
TMJ Fellow, Faculty of Medicine and Dentistry, University of Alberta, Edmonton, Alberta, Canada; Consultant, King Faisal Specialist Hospital and Research Centre, Riyadh, Saudi Arabia

JONATHAN BENSING, DMD, ML
Surgeon, Department of Oral and Maxillofacial Surgery, Walter Reed National Military Medical Center, Bethesda, Maryland, USA

BRIANA J. BURRIS, DDS, FACS
Program Director, Oral and Maxillofacial Surgery Residency Training Program, Department of Oral and Maxillofacial Surgery, Massachusetts General Hospital, Instructor, Harvard Medical School and Harvard School of Dental Medicine, Boston, Massachusetts, USA

BRIAN R. CARR, MD, DMD
Private Practice, Oral Surgery Associates of Milwaukee, Whitefish Bay, Wisconsin, USA

DAVID JOEY CHANG, DMD, FACS
Senior Clinical Instructor, Oral and Maxillofacial Surgery, Tufts University, Boston, Massachusetts, USA

DANIEL CHOI, DDS, MD, FACS
Assistant Director of Endoscopic Maxillofacial Surgery, Oral and Maxillofacial Surgery, Massachusetts General Hospital, Boston, Massachusetts, USA

JORDAN CIMILLUCA, DDS
Resident, Department of Oral and Maxillofacial Surgery, Uniformed Services University, Walter Reed National Military Medical Center, Bethesda, Maryland, USA

CLAYTON M. DAVIS, DDS, MD, MSc, FRCD(C)
Surgeon, Faculty of Medicine and Dentistry, University of Alberta, Kingsway Oral Maxillofacial Surgery, Edmonton, Alberta, Canada

ADIT GADH, DMD
Fellow, Endoscopic Maxillofacial Surgery, Oral and Maxillofacial Surgery, Massachusetts General Hospital, Boston, Massachusetts, USA

JEFFREY HAJIBANDEH, DDS, MD, FACS
Assistant Professor, Harvard Medical School and Harvard School of Dental Medicine, Medical Director of Quality, Oral and Maxillofacial Surgery, Oral Medicine, and Dentistry, Massachusetts General Hospital, Boston, Massachusetts, USA

MOHAMED HAKIM, DDS, MBA
Founder and Medical Director, Department of Oral and Maxillofacial Surgery, The International Center for TMJ and Jaw Surgery, Arlington, Virginia, USA

HANNAH JEFFRESS-VANDERS, DDS
Resident, Department of Oral and Maxillofacial Surgery, Uniformed Services University, Walter Reed National Military Medical Center, Bethesda, Maryland, USA

JAMIE LARMIE, MD, DDS
Resident, Department of Oral and Maxillofacial Surgery, UCLA School of Dentistry, Los Angeles, California, USA

JOSEPH P. McCAIN, DMD, FACS
Director of Endoscopic Maxillofacial Surgery, Department of Oral and Maxillofacial Surgery, Massachusetts General Hospital, Boston, Massachusetts, USA

JOHN M. SANDS, MD, DMD
Attending Physician, Department of Oral and Maxillofacial Surgery, Guthrie Hospital, Pennsylvania, USA

REBEKA SILVA, DMD, FACD
Chief, Division of Dental Service, Department of Oral and Maxillofacial Surgery, San Francisco VA Medical Center, San Francisco, California, USA

GABRIELLA TEHRANY, MD, DDS, FACS
Southern California Regional Chief, Department of Maxillofacial Surgery, Kaiser Sunset Los Angeles Medical Center, California, USA

GARY WARBURTON, DDS, MD, FDSRCS, FACS
Professor and Chair, Department of Oral and Maxillofacial Surgery, University of Maryland School of Dentistry, Baltimore, Maryland, USA

JULIAN WILSON, DDS, FACS
Attending Surgeon, Department of Oral and Maxillofacial Surgery, Kaiser Permanente, Instructor, University of California and Harbor-UCLA Medical Center, Los Angeles, California, USA

DAANESH ZAKAI, MBChB, BDS
Fellow, Department of Pediatric Craniomaxillofacial Surgery, Great Ormond Street Hospital, London, United Kingdom

Contents

ATLAS OF THE ORAL AND MAXILLOFACIAL SURGERY CLINICS OF NORTH AMERICA

FORTHCOMING ISSUES

March 2027

Step-by-Step Approach to AI-Guided Surgical Planning
Fernando P.S. Guastaldi, Balazs Feher and Zachary S. Peacock, *Editors*

September 2027

Peripheral Nerve Reconstruction in the Head and Neck
Marina Morante Silva, *Editor*

RECENT ISSUES

March 2026

Implant Solutions for Complex Cases with Grafting
Vishtasb Broumand, *Editor*

September 2025

Implant Solutions for Complex Cases: Graftless Solutions
Vishtasb Broumand, *Editor*

March 2025

Maxillary and Midface Reconstruction, Part 2
Michael R. Markiewicz, James C. Melville, and Rui P. Fernandes, *Editors*

Preface

The Temporomandibular Joint: An Operative Atlas from Arthrocentesis to Total Joint Reconstruction

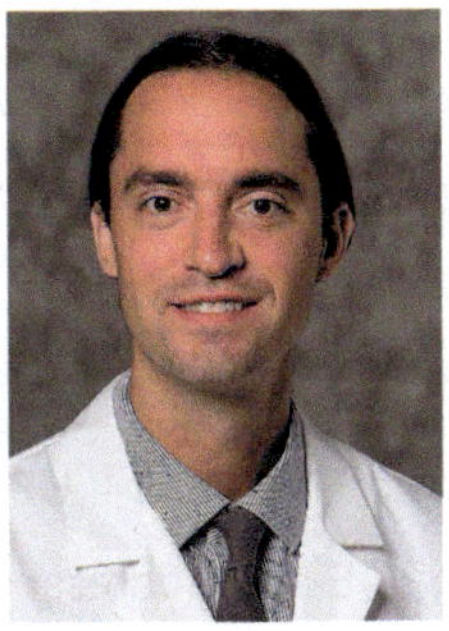

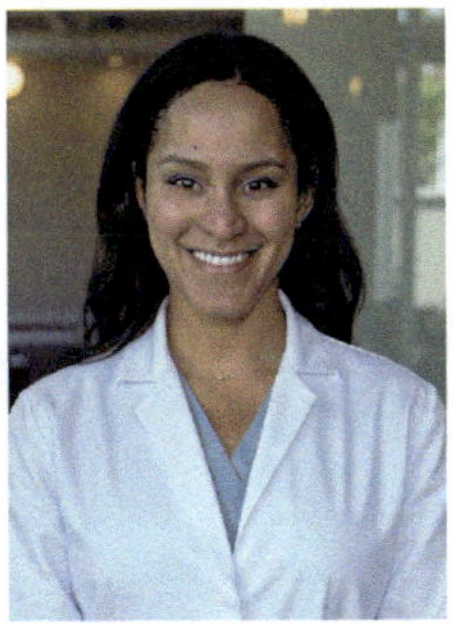

Daniel P. Caruso, MD, DDS   Briana J. Burris, DDS, FACS

Editors

Temporomandibular joint (TMJ) surgery spans one of the widest operative ranges within oral and maxillofacial surgery. Few anatomic regions demand such fluency across interventions—from needle-based intra-articular therapy, to arthroscopic visualization, to open joint reconstruction, to alloplastic total joint replacement combined with orthognathic correction. The region is unforgiving of imprecision, and it has evolved rapidly over the past decade through the integration of virtual surgical planning, custom prosthesis design, and increasingly defined indications for staged and combined procedures.

This issue of the *Atlas of the Oral and Maxillofacial Surgery Clinics of North America* is built to function as an operative reference rather than a narrative review. Each article is procedure-driven: indications and contraindications are stated explicitly; surgical anatomy is presented with operative relevance; and technique is taught in stepwise sequence with instrument-level detail, anatomic plane transitions, and verification endpoints. Decision making is rendered as an algorithm where appropriate. Complications are addressed both within individual articles and as a dedicated article on revision and salvage. The intent is an issue that the trainee can study before a case and the experienced surgeon can consult at the operative table.

The issue opens with TMJ imaging and surgical anatomy, establishing the radiographic and three-dimensional foundation on which every subsequent procedure depends. The minimally invasive continuum is addressed through arthrocentesis, intra-articular injection, and diagnostic and operative arthroscopy, with emphasis on portal placement, endoscopic anatomy, and reproducible technical endpoints. Open joint surgery—arthroplasty, discectomy, disc repositioning, and eminectomy—is presented with attention to exposure, disc handling, graft selection, and intraoperative decision making.

Atlas Oral Maxillofacial Surg Clin N Am 34 (2026) xi–xii
1061-3315/26/© 2026 Published by Elsevier Inc.
https://doi.org/10.1016/j.cxom.2026.05.009

Subsequent articles extend this operative framework to ankylosis, autogenous and alloplastic reconstruction, TMJ pathologic condition, combined TMJ–orthognathic surgery, complications, revision surgery, and rehabilitation.

TMJ surgery is no longer a discrete subspecialty of last resort but a defined continuum of staged interventions, each with explicit indications, reproducible technique, and measurable outcomes. The contributors to this issue are surgeons who operate at every point along that continuum, and the articles reflect what they actually do in the operating room. Our hope is that this issue is returned to before cases rather than read once and shelved.

We thank the contributing authors for their expertise, our developmental editorial team at Elsevier for their support, and our families for their patience.

Disclosures

Dr D.P. Caruso has no commercial or financial relationships and no funding sources to disclose. Dr B.J. Burris has no commercial or financial relationships and no funding sources to disclose.

Daniel P. Caruso, MD, DDS
Department of Oral and
Maxillofacial Surgery
Division of Head and Neck Surgery
University of Florida College
of Medicine–Jacksonville
653-1 West 8th Street
Jacksonville, FL 32209, USA

Briana J. Burris, DDS, FACS
Division of Oral and
Maxillofacial Surgery
Massachusetts General Hospital
55 Fruit Street
Boston, MA 02114, USA

E-mail addresses:
daniel.caruso@jax.ufl.edu (D.P. Caruso)
bburris@mgh.harvard.edu (B.J. Burris)

Temporomandibular Joint Imaging and Surgical Anatomy

John M. Sands, MD, DMD [a,*], Brian R. Carr, MD, DMD [b]

KEYWORDS

• Temporomandibular joint (TMJ) • Internal derangement (ID) • Degenerative joint disease (DJD) • MRI • Surgical anatomy

KEY POINTS

- The temporomandibular joint (TMJ) is a unique load-bearing synovial joint with fibrocartilage surfaces, adapted for repetitive functional stress.
- Internal derangement and degenerative joint disease are the most common TMJ pathologies and often coexist with progressive changes.
- Imaging is essential for diagnosis, with MRI as the gold standard for soft tissues and computed tomography (CT)/cone-beam computed tomography (CBCT) for osseous evaluation.
- TMJ disorders are multifactorial, involving mechanical overload, anatomy, and adaptive capacity, with structural changes sometimes present in asymptomatic individuals.
- Understanding surgical anatomy, including vascular and neural relationships, is critical for safe intervention and optimal outcomes.

Etiologic considerations

Temporomandibular joint (TMJ) disorders are multifactorial.[1] Internal derangement (ID)—an abnormal positional relationship between the disc, condyle, and articular eminence—has been reported in up to 70% of symptomatic patients[2] and is commonly staged using the Wilkes system (Stages I–V), which links progressive disc displacement to escalating pain and structural damage.[3] Degenerative joint disease (DJD) is typically noninflammatory and characterized by cartilage deterioration, subchondral remodeling, osteophyte formation, and secondary synovitis. Mechanical overload from trauma, parafunction, occlusal instability, and repetitive loading may exceed the adaptive capacity of the disc and retrodiscal tissues. Structural abnormalities are present in approximately 25% of asymptomatic individuals,[4] which establishes a critical surgical principle: imaging findings must be correlated with clinical examination before they drive operative decisions.

Osseous temporomandibular joint anatomy

The TMJ is a ginglymoarthrodial articulation formed by the mandibular condyle and the temporal bone—specifically the glenoid fossa and articular eminence (Fig. 1).[5] The temporal component comprises the glenoid fossa posteriorly and the articular eminence anteriorly (Figs. 2 and 3). The glenoid fossa is bounded posteriorly by the tympanic plate and anteriorly by the articular tubercle. Mean glenoid fossa depth is 7.5 mm and mean articular eminence inclination is 49.9°.[6] The roof of the glenoid fossa is notably thin (mean ~0.9 mm)[7]—a surgically relevant threshold given that this bone separates the joint from the middle cranial fossa during arthroscopic puncture and elevator instrumentation. Steeper eminence inclinations increase translational demands on the disc-condyle complex and are associated with greater disc displacement severity; flatter eminences predispose to posterior condylar positioning and altered loading.[8,9]

Normal condylar morphology is characterized by a smooth cortical outline with trabecular bone oriented along principal stress trajectories (Figs. 4 and 5).[10] Cortical thinning, surface flattening, and trabecular disorganization may represent adaptive remodeling rather than frank pathology[11]; osteophyte formation, subchondral sclerosis, and contour change likewise occur in asymptomatic individuals.[12] The surgical implications are twofold: preoperative CT or CBCT should define the relationship of the fossa roof to planned arthroscopic trajectories, and condylar morphology must inform prosthesis fit and screw-purchase planning in alloplastic reconstruction.

Disc and soft-tissue anatomy

The articular disc is a biconcave fibrocartilaginous structure interposed between the condyle and the temporal component (Fig. 6). The disc is composed of dense collagen with regional thickness variation—approximately 3 mm posteriorly, 1 mm in the intermediate zone, and 2 mm anteriorly[13,14]—and is relatively avascular and aneural. The bilaminar (retrodiscal) zone is highly vascularized and innervated, containing elastic fibers that permit anterior disc translation during mandibular movement.[15,16]

[a] Department of Oral & Maxillofacial Surgery, Guthrie Hospital, PA, USA
[b] Private Practice, Oral Surgery Associates, Whitefish Bay, WI, USA
* Corresponding author.
E-mail address: john@goaroms.com

Atlas Oral Maxillofacial Surg Clin N Am 34 (2026) 185-199

https://doi.org/10.1016/j.cxom.2026.05.001
oralmaxsurgeryatlas.theclinics.com

Abbreviations

DJD degenerative joint disease
ID internal derangement
TMJ temporomandibular joint

MRI is the standard for evaluation of disc position, morphology, and associated soft-tissue pathology (Figs. 7–9). Disc displacement is classically categorized as anterior displacement with or without reduction, based on the disc-condyle relationship in closed- and open-mouth positions.[14] Displacement severity correlates with joint effusion, retrodiscal inflammation, and disease progression, although displacement alone does not reliably predict symptom severity (Fig. 10).[17] Inflammatory change within the retrodiscal tissues—rather than disc position itself—appears to be the primary pain generator in many patients (Fig. 11). These distinctions are operatively decisive: isolated displacement without effusion or retrodiscal signal change favors arthroscopic lysis and lavage; effusion plus retrodiscal inflammation supports arthroscopy with disc repositioning; a deformed, perforated disc with advanced DJD favors discectomy or alloplastic reconstruction.

Capsule and ligaments

The TMJ capsule encloses the joint and contributes to stability, proprioception, and synovial fluid containment, with sensory innervation that mediates joint position sense and pain.[18] Capsular distention—visualized on MRI as joint effusion or synovitis—correlates with arthralgia and functional limitation. Collateral ligaments anchor the medial and lateral disc margins to the condyle, ensuring coordinated disc-condyle motion; the temporomandibular, sphenomandibular, and stylomandibular ligaments provide secondary restraint (Fig. 12). Ligamentous structures themselves are inconsistently visualized on MRI.[19]

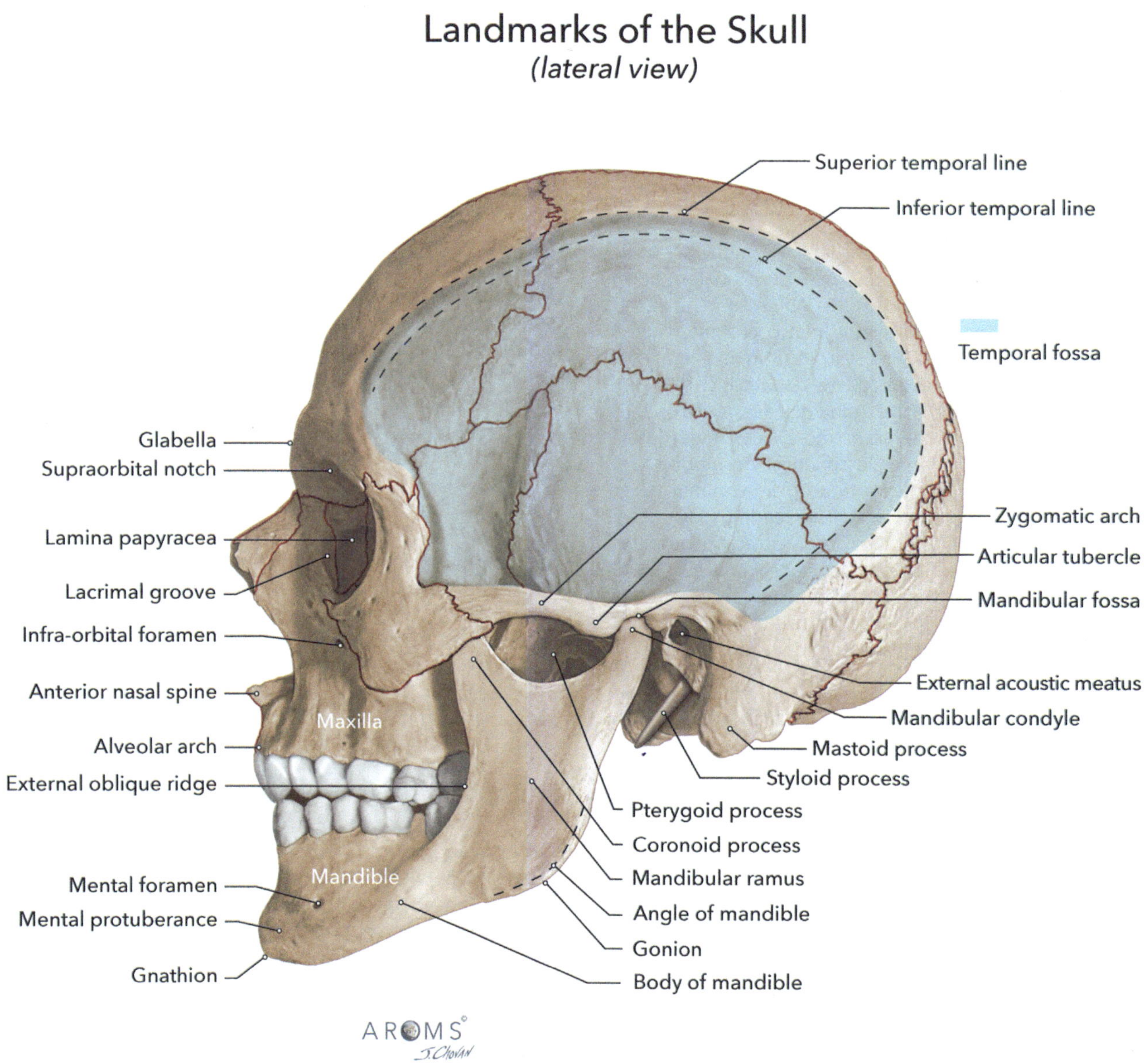

Fig. 1 Anatomic landmarks of the skull.

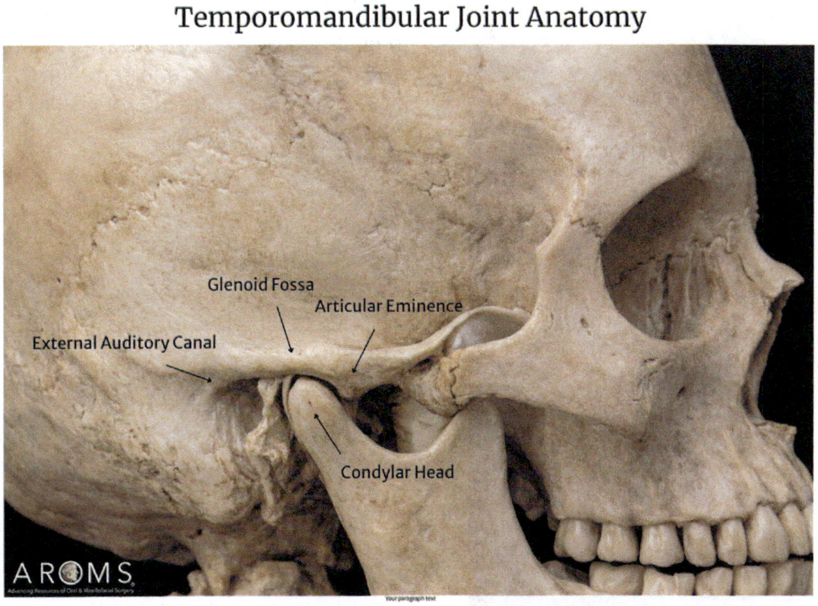

Fig. 2 TMJ osseous anatomy sagittal view.

Vascular anatomy and surgical danger zones

The medial aspect of the TMJ is a zone of heightened surgical risk: major neurovascular structures may lie within millimeters of the medial capsule. The *rule of 2s* provides a practical framework—the lateral capsule lies approximately 2 cm from the skin, the medial capsule approximately 2 cm medial to the lateral capsule, and major vascular and neural structures approximately 2 cm medial to the medial capsule.[5]

Vascular anatomy is highly variable. The maxillary artery may course medial or lateral to the lateral pterygoid muscle (Fig. 13); its branches—masseteric, deep temporal, and middle meningeal—contribute to the periarticular blood supply (Fig. 14). Quantitative cadaveric and angiographic data establish the working distances: the middle meningeal artery averages 19 mm from the condylar apex and 15 mm from the medial condylar point, the maxillary artery lies within 6 to 7 mm of the sigmoid notch,[20] and the masseteric artery may be as little as 4 mm from the condylar neck, 3 mm from the articular tubercle, and 1 mm from the sigmoid notch.[21] Venous

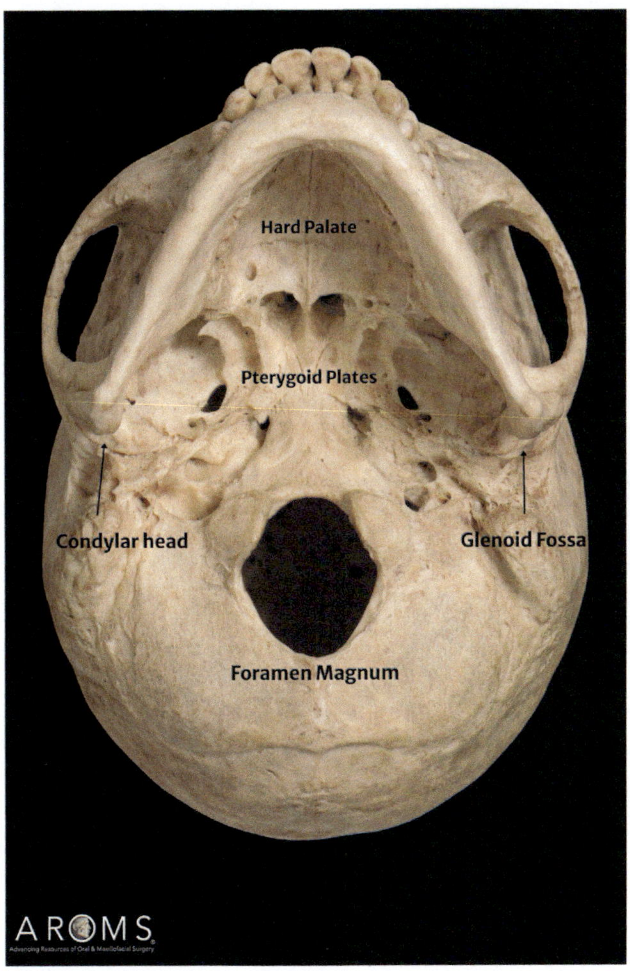

Fig. 3 TMJ osseous anatomy axial view.

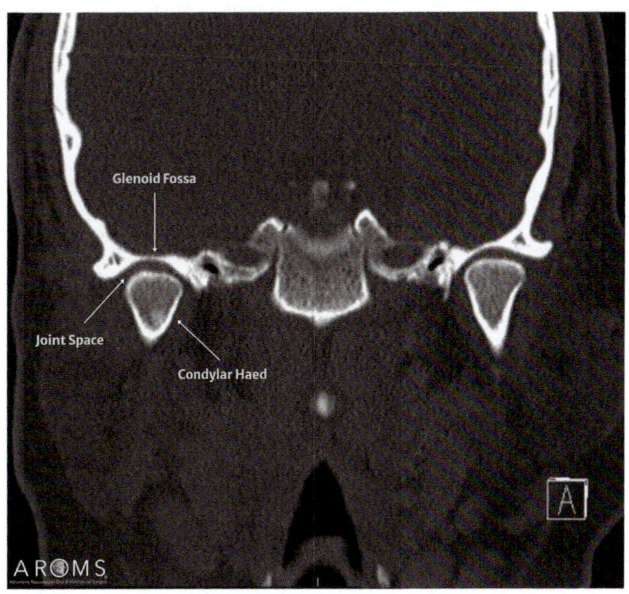

Fig. 4 CT of normal condylar morphology coronal view.

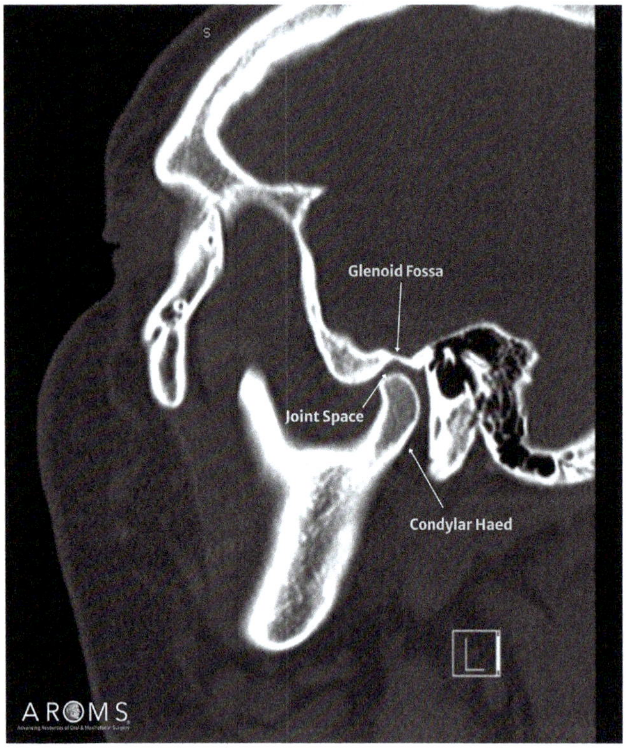

Fig. 5 CT of normal condylar morphology sagittal view.

drainage occurs primarily through the pterygoid venous plexus (Fig. 15),[22] a low-pressure, high-volume bleeding source difficult to control once entered. Superficial temporal vessels are at risk during preauricular incision. CT angiography is useful in revision and complex cases for defining vascular relationships before incision.[23]

Neural anatomy

Sensory innervation of the TMJ is primarily from the auriculotemporal nerve, a branch of V3. The nerve courses posterior and medial to the condylar neck and frequently contacts the capsule and posterior discal tissues, providing an anatomic basis for referred otologic and temporal pain. Entrapment by inflamed retrodiscal tissues has been proposed as a mechanism in TMJ pain syndromes.[24]

The temporal branch of the facial nerve is the principal motor structure at risk during open TMJ approaches. Cadaveric studies place this branch within 3 to 10 mm of the lateral condylar pole and crossing the zygomatic arch between 8 to 35 mm anterior to the bony external acoustic meatus (Fig. 16).[25] Imaging cannot reliably visualize the nerve; protection is achieved surgically by dissecting deep to the superficial layer of the deep temporal fascia above the arch, minimizing anterior retraction, and avoiding electrocautery within the danger zone (Figs. 17 and 18).

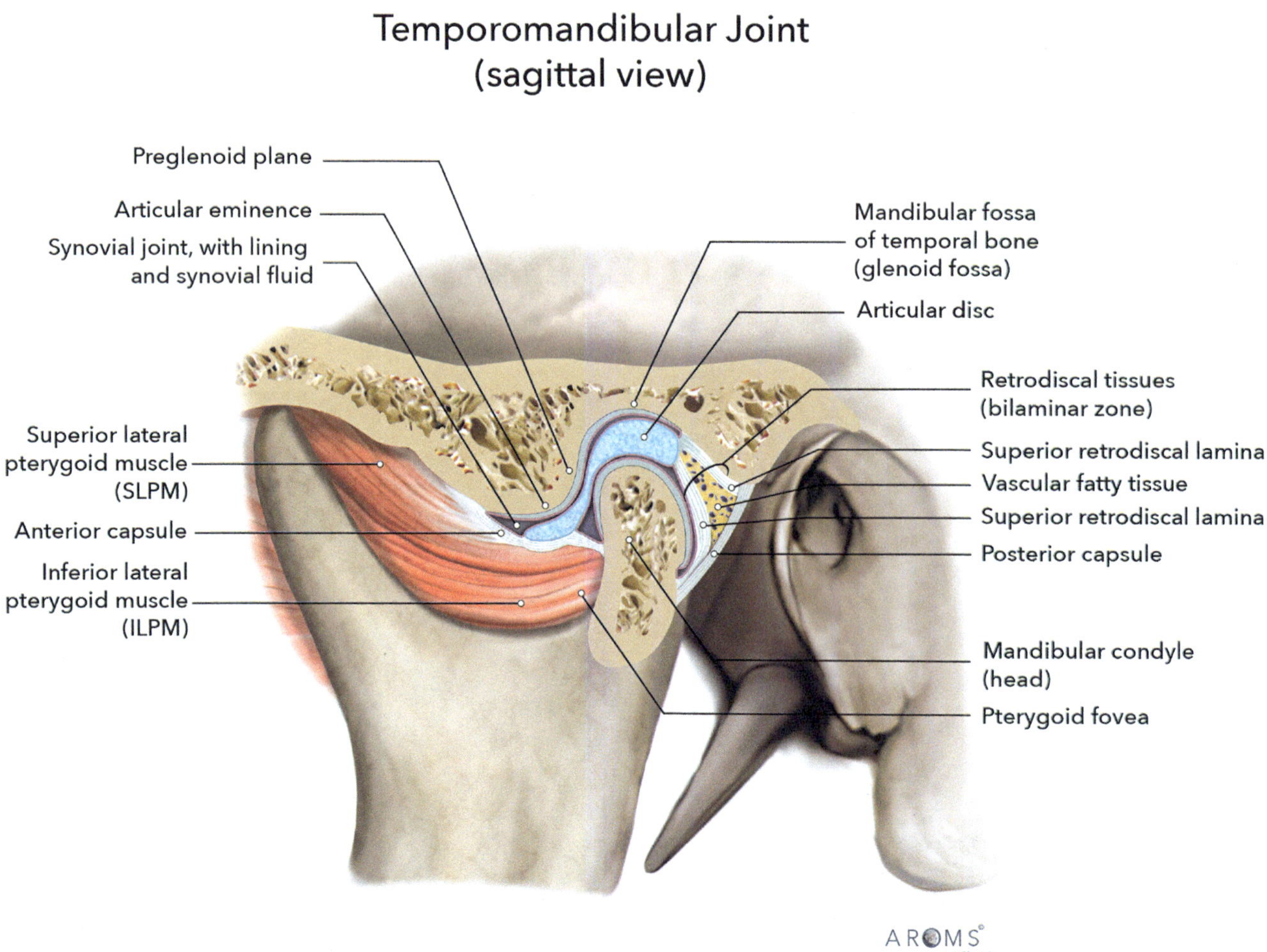

Fig. 6 Normal TMJ soft Tissue and disc anatomy.

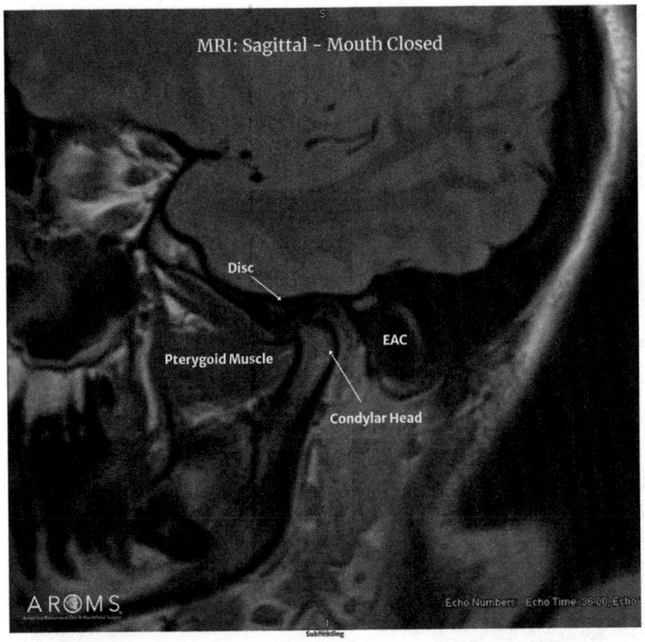

Fig. 7 T1 weighted MRI showing normal disc position, sagittal view closed mouth.

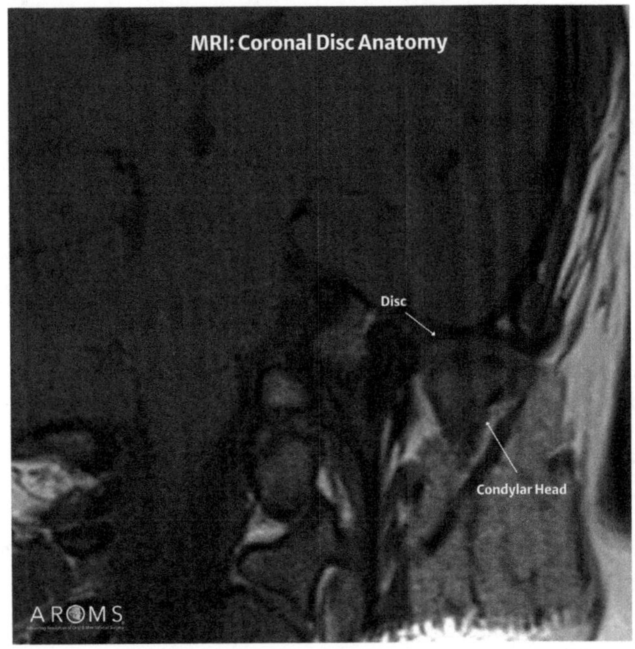

Fig. 9 T1 weighted MRI showing normal disc position, coronal view closed mouth.

Imaging modalities in temporomandibular joint evaluation

Clinical examination alone has poor agreement with imaging-confirmed ID or osteoarthritis,[26] so imaging is typically required to establish the presence, severity, and extent of intra-articular disease (Table 1).

Panoramic radiography and CBCT

Panoramic radiography and CBCT serve as accessible screening tools, particularly for gross osseous morphology and asymmetry. CBCT offers superior spatial resolution compared with panoramic imaging at a lower dose than conventional CT, but both are limited in soft-tissue assessment (Table 2).[27]

Computed tomography

Conventional CT remains the standard for complex osseous pathology—fractures, ankylosis, heterotopic bone, and advanced DJD—and provides critical information for open joint surgery and total joint replacement, including condylar measurements and screw-trajectory planning.

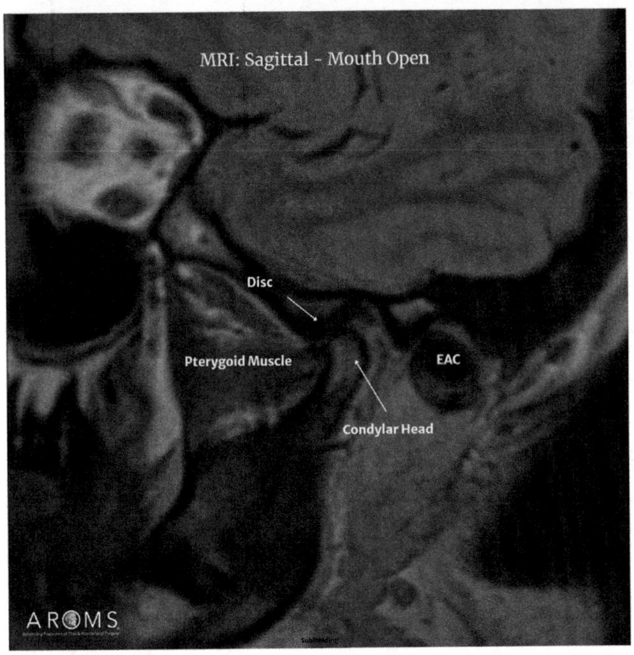

Fig. 8 T1 weighted MRI showing normal disc position, sagittal view open mouth.

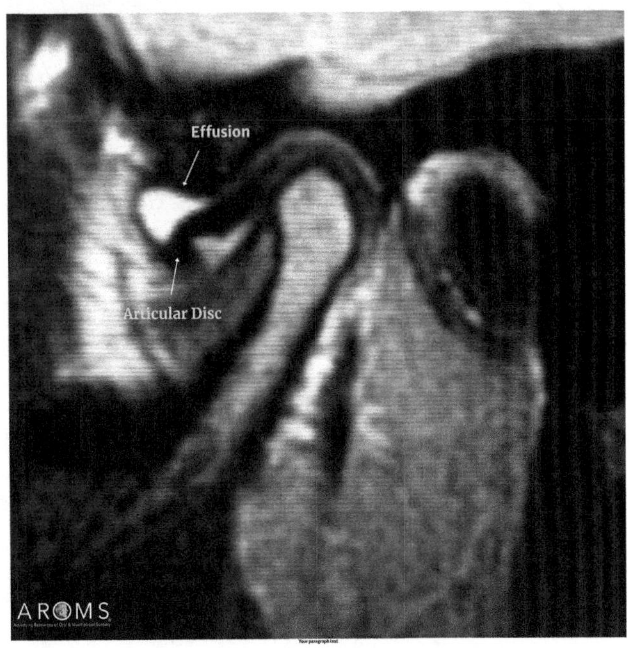

Fig. 10 T2 weighted MRI showing joint effusion, sagittal view.

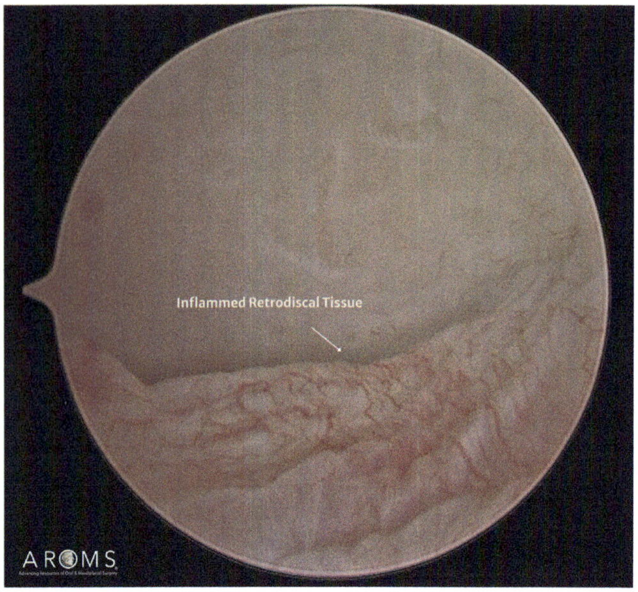

Fig. 11 Arthroscopy showing inflamed retrodiscal Tissue.

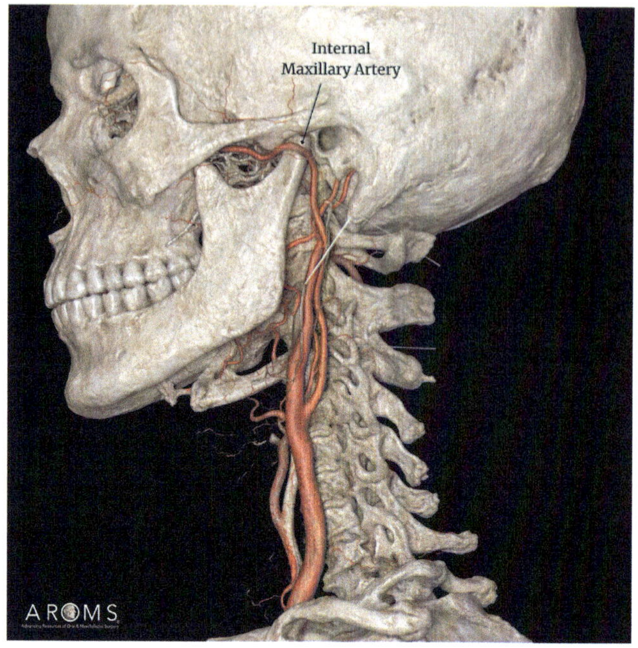

Fig. 13 Internal maxillary artery relationship to the condylar neck.

Magnetic resonance imaging

MRI is the standard for disc position, joint effusion, marrow edema, and synovitis, and is warranted in therapy-resistant cases, suspected ID, and surgical planning. Dynamic MRI further improves diagnostic accuracy and correlates more closely with arthroscopic findings than static sequences.[28] Two methods are used to assess disc position: the traditional *12-o'clock* method and the intermediate zone method.[29] The

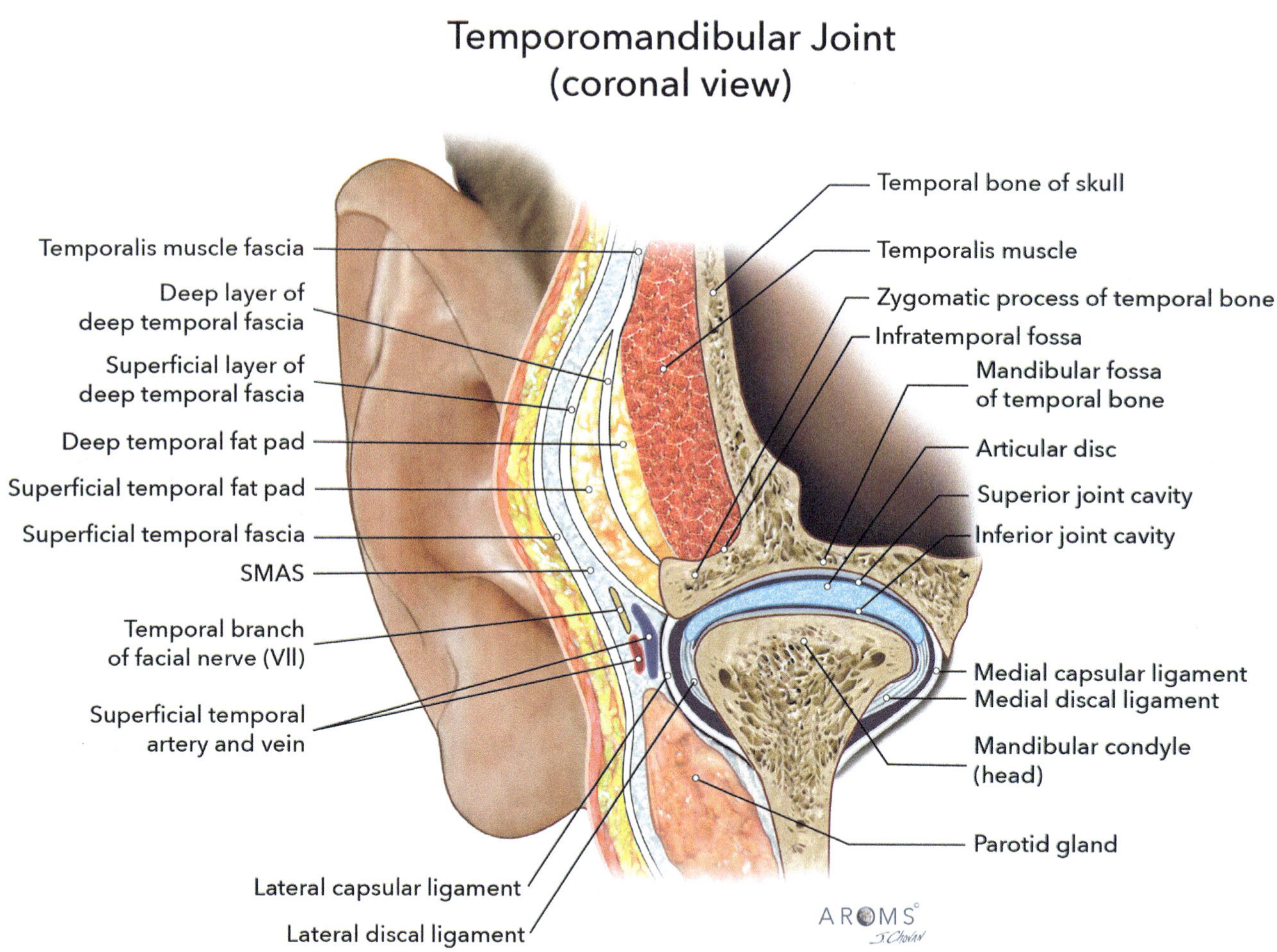

Fig. 12 Collateral and secondary ligaments of the TMJ.

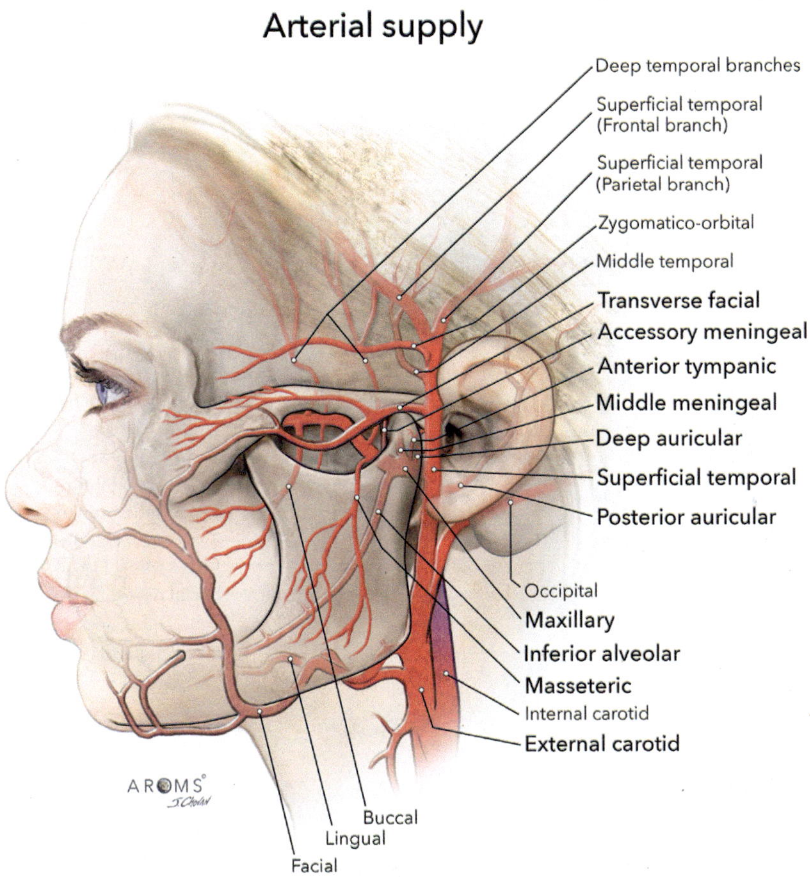

Fig. 14 Arterial supply of the TMJ.

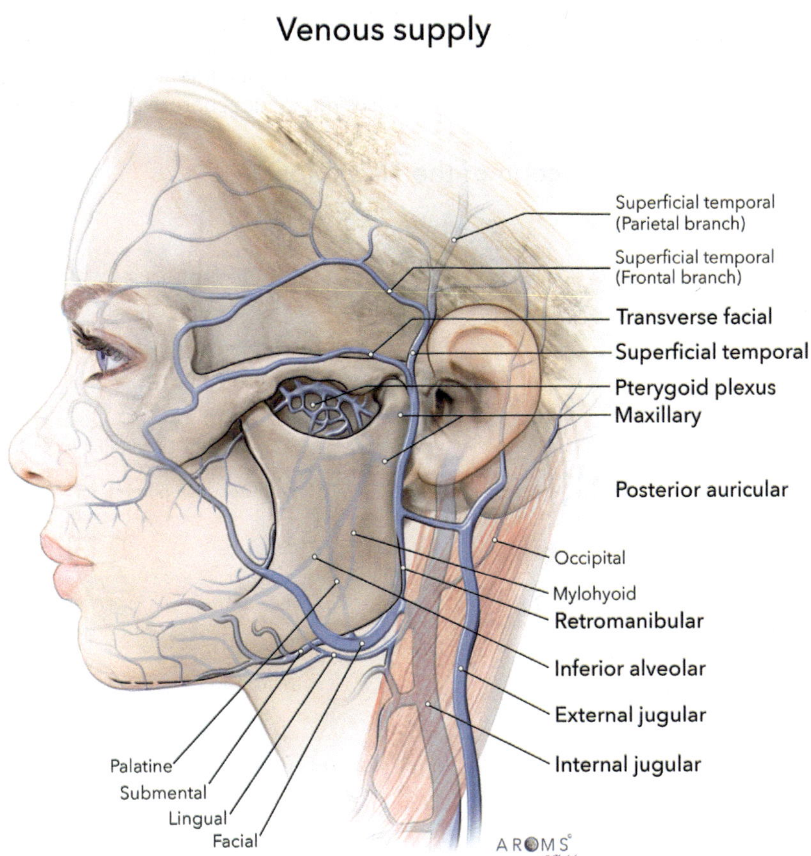

Fig. 15 Venous drainage of the TMJ.

Facial Nerve: Temporal Branch

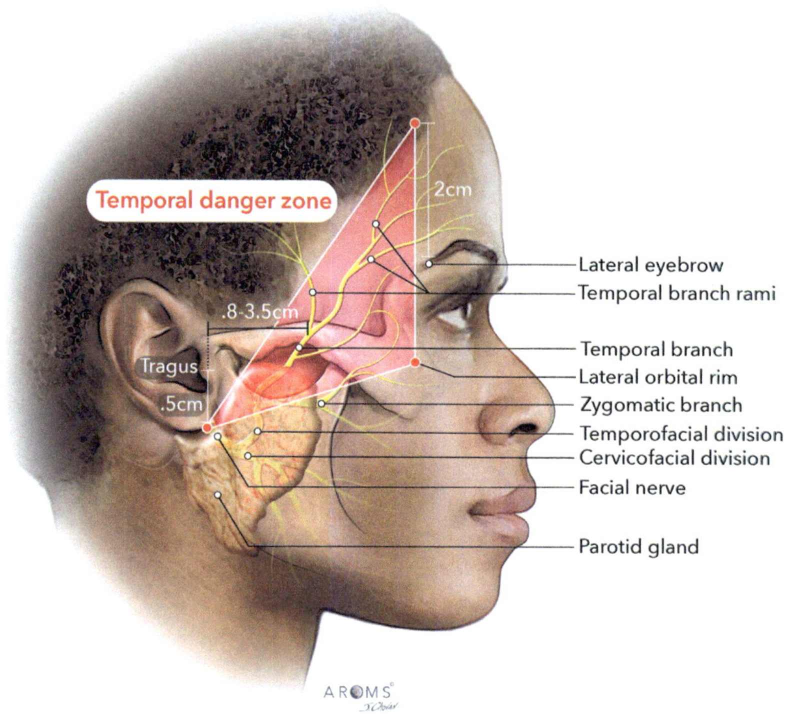

Fig. 16 Anatomy of the temporal branch of the facial nerve.

12-o'clock method overdiagnoses anterior displacement and yields high false-positive rates in asymptomatic subjects; the intermediate zone method—evaluating the functional relationship between intermediate zone, condylar head, and articular eminence—demonstrates superior sensitivity, specificity, and clinical correlation (Figs. 19 and 20). The choice of method matters operatively: a 12-o'clock *displacement* in an asymptomatic joint should not, on its own, drive a surgical recommendation.

MRI findings correlate with clinical severity.[30] Progressive anterior displacement is associated with increasing joint effusion, degenerative osseous change, retrodiscal

Dissection of the TMJ Capsule

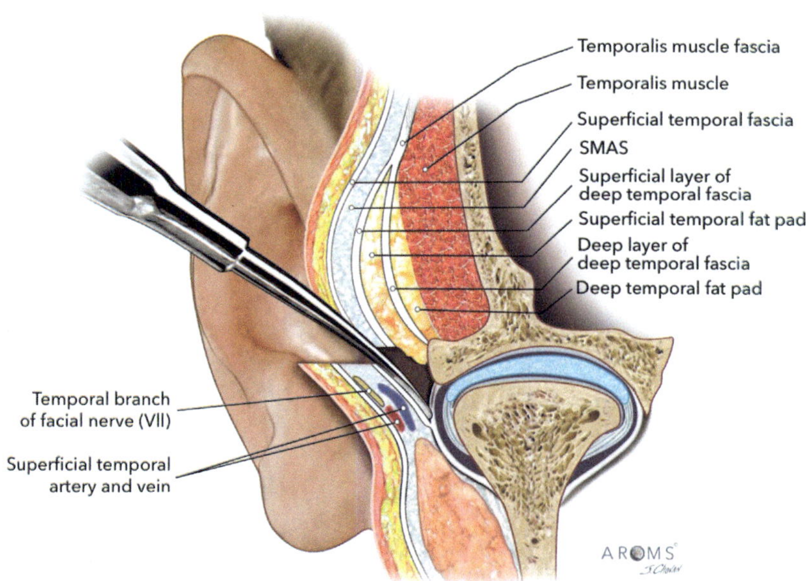

Fig. 17 Surgical dissection of the TMJ capsule.

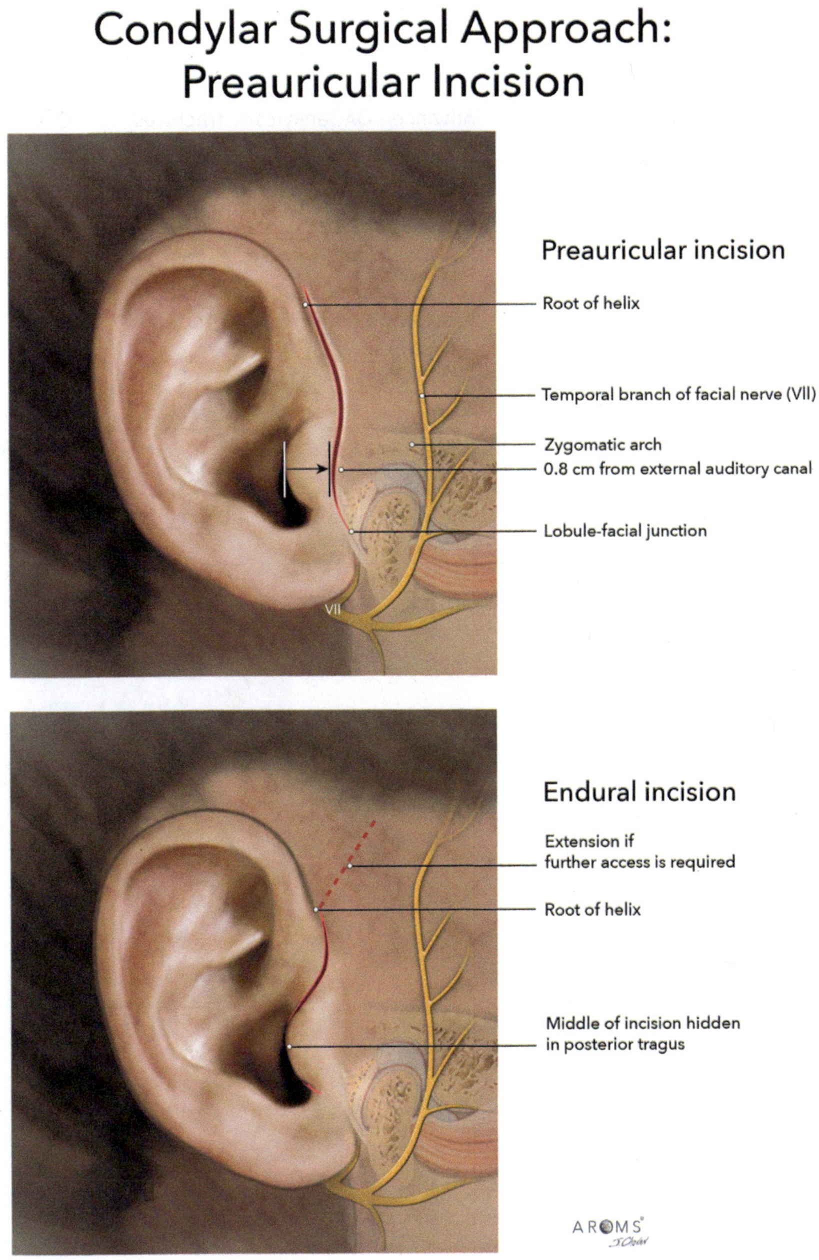

Fig. 18 Preauricular and endaural incision designs.

Table 1 Imaging modality strengths and limitations

Modality	Best for	Strengths	Limitations
Panorex	Initial screening	Fast, cheap, widely available; gross condylar morphology, asymmetry, fractures, advanced osteoarthritis (OA)	Poor TMJ detail; 2D distortion; cannot assess disc, effusion, and synovitis
MRI	Soft tissue/TMJ internal derangement (IPD)	Gold standard for disc position/morphology, effusion, synovitis, retrodiscal inflammation, and marrow edema	Limited bony detail; costly; motion artifact; longer study time
CT	Osseous disease/advanced OA	Best for erosions, osteophytes, sclerosis, ankylosis, fractures; excellent for surgical planning/TJR workup	Radiation; limited soft tissue evaluation
CBCT	Outpatient bony evaluation	High bony resolution with lower radiation than CT; excellent condyle/fossa remodeling, OA changes	Cannot evaluate disc or inflammation; less ideal for complex reconstruction planning than CT

Table 2 Comparative table for imaging modalities

Feature	MRI	CT (Medical-Grade)	CBCT
Primary Strength	Soft tissue + inflammation	High-resolution bone imaging	High-resolution bone imaging (low dose)
Best For	Disc pathology, synovitis, effusion, IPD	Advanced OA, ankylosis, fractures, TJR planning	Outpatient evaluation of bony remodeling/OA
Disc Evaluation	Excellent (gold standard)	Poor	Poor
Synovitis/Effusion	Excellent	Limited	Not visualized
Osseous Degeneration (OA)	Moderate (secondary changes only)	Excellent (gold standard)	Excellent
Surgical Planning Utility	Helpful for soft tissue planning	*Best for complex cases/total joint replacement (TJR)*	Good for bony planning, less ideal for complex reconstruction
Radiation	None	Moderate	Low (relative to CT)
Cost/Access	Higher cost, limited access	Moderate–high	Moderate, widely available in dental settings
Key Limitation	Weak bony detail and motion artifact	Cannot evaluate disc/inflammation well	No soft tissue/inflammatory information

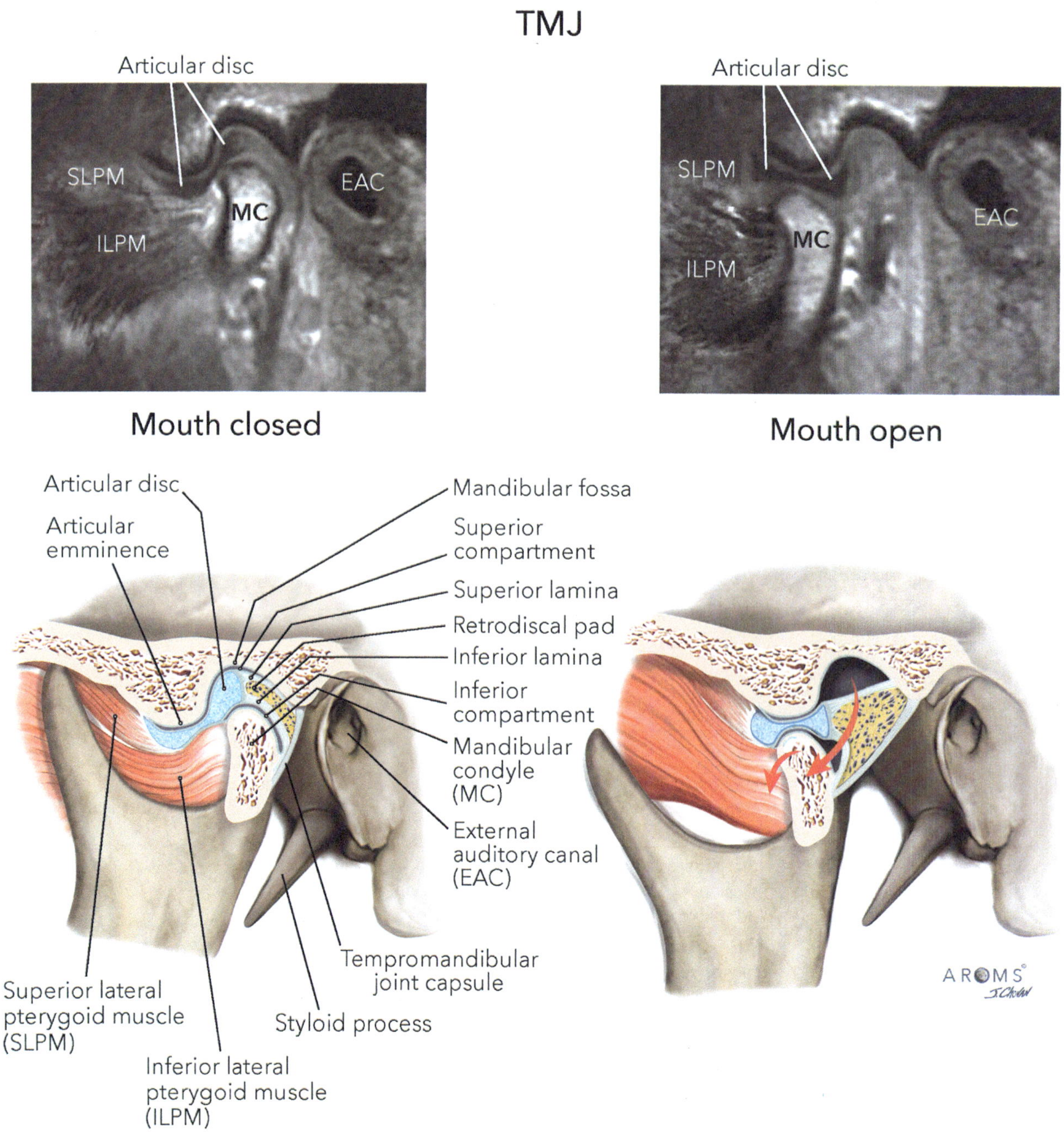

Fig. 19 Correlation between MRI of the TMJ and clinical anatomy.

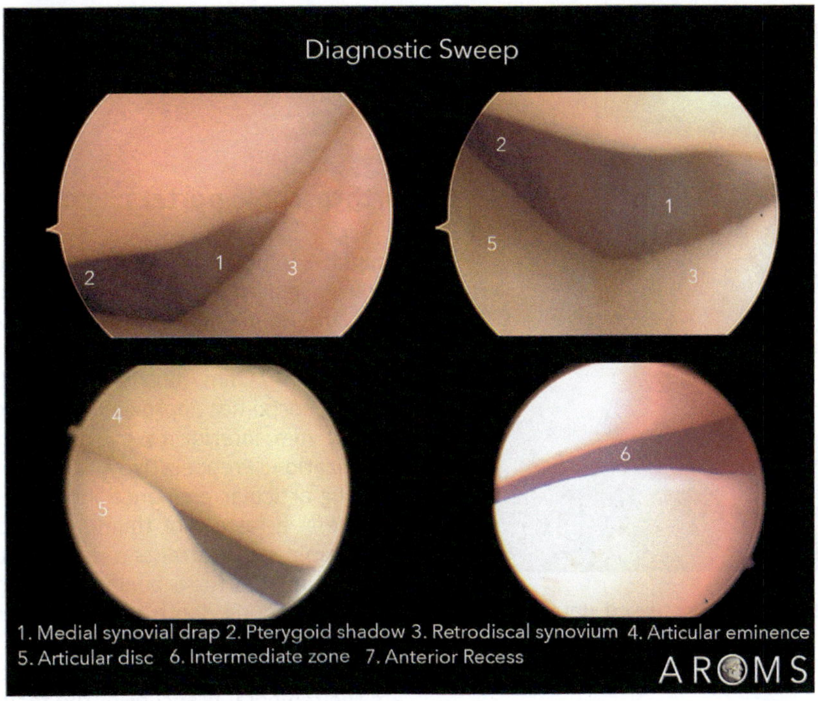

Fig. 20 Arthroscopic anatomy of the TMJ: Medial synovial drape, retrodiscal synovium, articular eminence, articular disc, intermediate zone, anterior recess.

abnormalities, and lateral pterygoid alterations (Figs. 21 and 22). Joint effusion correlates with arthralgia severity and decreased maximal incisal opening and serves as an imaging marker of active intra-articular inflammation.

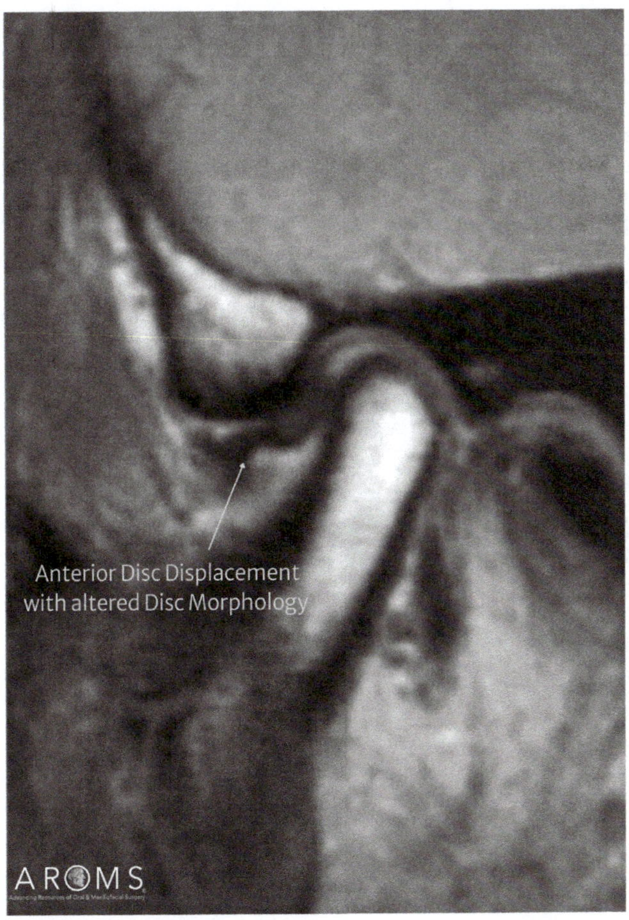

Fig. 21 T1 weighted MRI showing anterior disc displacement with altered disc morphology, sagittal view closed mouth.

Nuclear medicine

Technetium-99m bone scintigraphy and single photon emission computed tomography (SPECT)/CT identify metabolically active condylar growth or inflammation, particularly in facial asymmetry or suspected condylar hyperplasia (Fig. 23).[31,32] Interpretation requires caution because inflammatory TMJ disease can yield false positives.

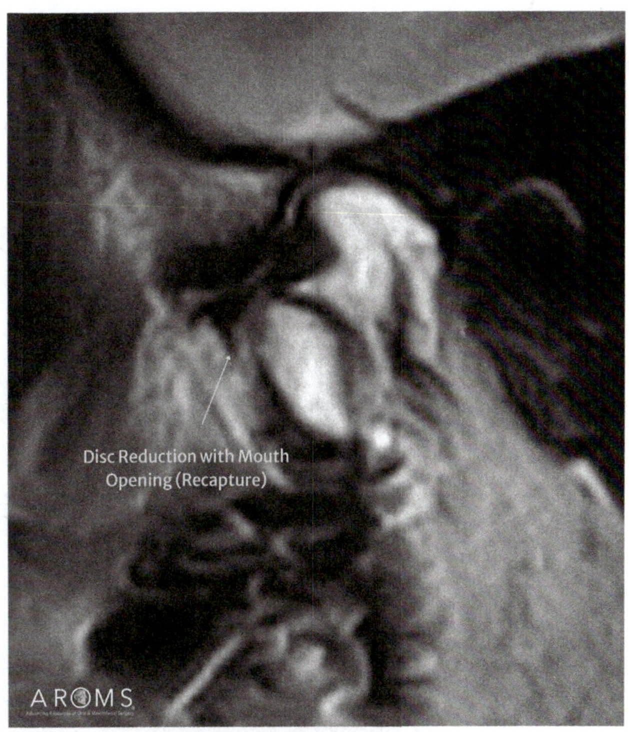

Fig. 22 T1 weighted MRI showing disc recapture in the open mouth view (anterior disc displacement with reduction), sagittal view.

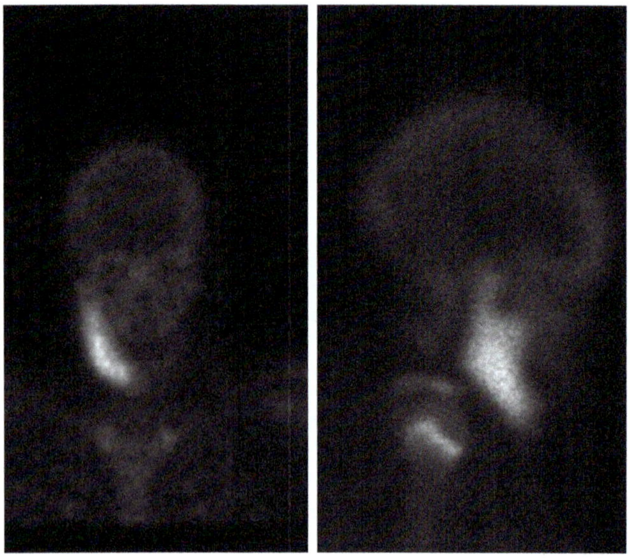

Fig. 23 Technetium-99 scan showing increased uptake in the right ramus and condylar region.

Three-dimensional reconstruction and virtual surgical planning

Three-dimensional imaging and virtual surgical planning enable volumetric assessment of condylar morphology, objective asymmetry analysis, and improved surgical accuracy through patient-specific guides and prostheses. These workflows are increasingly integrated into TMJ reconstruction and hold promise for outcome prediction and precision surgery (Figs. 24 and 25).[33,34] Overall, modality selection should be driven by the specific anatomic and surgical question; an actionable decision framework is presented in Table 3.

Surgical approaches: anatomic and imaging correlation

While dedicated technique articles address each procedure in detail, the following framework links the imaging and anatomy reviewed earlier to the 2 approaches most relevant to TMJ surgery: arthroscopic portal placement and the preauricular open approach. Critical working distances are consolidated in Table 4.

Arthroscopic portal placement

Standard arthroscopic access uses 2 portals into the superior joint space. The posterolateral (initial) puncture is established along the Holmlund-Hellsing line drawn from the tragus to the lateral canthus: entry approximately 10 mm anterior to the tragus and 2 mm inferior to the line.[7] The anterolateral working portal lies approximately 20 mm anterior to the tragus and 10 mm inferior to the line, triangulated under direct visualization. Preoperative CBCT informs portal trajectory by defining articular eminence inclination and glenoid fossa roof thickness; a fossa roof thinner than the mean ~0.9 mm[7] or a steep eminence warrants a more posteriorly directed cannula to avoid middle fossa penetration, and steep eminences also increase working depth and may necessitate a more anterior anterolateral portal.

The principal danger structures along the portal trajectory are the temporal branches of the facial nerve superficially, the auriculotemporal nerve and superficial temporal vessels in the preauricular soft tissue, and the middle meningeal artery deep to the fossa roof. Strict adherence to the Holmlund-Hellsing line and an inferior-to-superior cannula direction protect these structures.

Preauricular approach

The modified preauricular (Al-Kayat-Bramley) approach remains the workhorse for open TMJ surgery.[25] The incision parallels the preauricular crease and may be extended superiorly in a question-mark fashion to expose the zygomatic arch. The key dissection plane is identified beneath the superficial layer of the deep temporal fascia, which is incised at a 45° angle from the root of the zygomatic arch toward the superior limit of the incision. Dissection then proceeds medially along the lateral surface of the temporalis fascia, deep to the temporal branch of the facial nerve, which lies within the

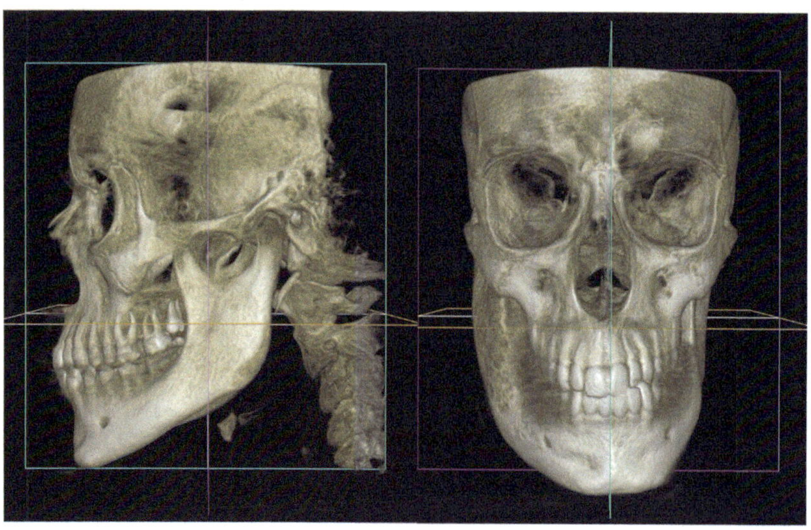

Fig. 24 3D reconstruction of osseous anatomy.

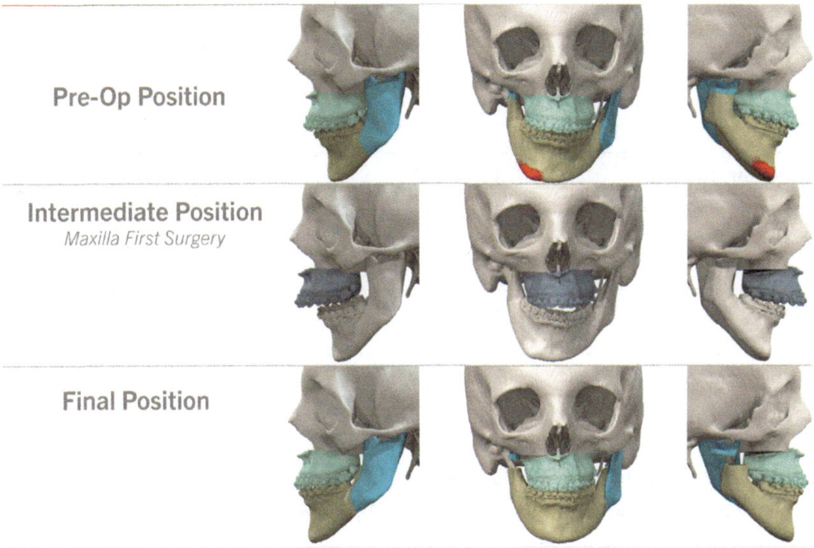

Fig. 25 Virtual surgical planning showing preop, intermediate, and final positions.

Table 3 Imaging decision framework for temporomandibular joint surgical planning

Clinical Scenario	Preferred Modality	Key Findings to Evaluate	Impact on Surgical Planning
Suspected internal derangement (mechanical symptoms, and locking)	MRI (closed and open mouth)	Disc position by intermediate zone method; effusion; retrodiscal signal change	Lysis/lavage vs disc repositioning vs discectomy
Persistent arthralgia, treatment-resistant	MRI + clinical correlation	Joint effusion; synovitis; marrow edema; lateral pterygoid signal	Confirms active inflammation as arthroscopy target
Trauma, fracture, and ankylosis	CT (high-resolution)	Fracture pattern; heterotopic bone; osseous fusion; condylar displacement	Open reduction, internal fixation (ORIF) planning; gap arthroplasty corridor; airway risk
Advanced DJD or planned alloplastic reconstruction	CT (with 3D reconstruction)	Condylar resorption; fossa morphology; screw-purchase bone stock	Patient-specific implant design; cutting and drilling guides
Facial asymmetry, suspected condylar hyperplasia	SPECT/CT + CBCT	Asymmetric condylar uptake; condylar morphology and height	Timing of condylectomy; need for orthognathic correction
Prearthroscopy screening	CBCT or panoramic	Osseous morphology; fossa roof thickness; and eminence inclination	Identifies steep eminences and thin fossa roof that alter portal trajectory
Revision surgery or anomalous anatomy	CT angiography	Maxillary, middle meningeal, and masseteric artery course	Defines vascular danger zone before incision

temporoparietal fascia 8 to 35 mm anterior to the bony external acoustic meatus.[25] The capsule is reached by sharp dissection along the lateral surface of the zygomatic arch and articular eminence.

Three danger zones require deliberate management. (1) Facial nerve: stay deep to the superficial layer of the deep temporal fascia and avoid anterior retraction beyond the lateral orbital rim. (2) Superficial temporal vessels: identify and retract or ligate before they restrict exposure. (3) Maxillary artery and pterygoid plexus: avoid medial capsular penetration; the *rule of 2s*[5] defines the working envelope, and CT angiography is indicated in revision cases or when imaging suggests anomalous vascular position. When entering the inferior joint space, preserve disc-condyle attachments medially to avoid traction on the auriculotemporal nerve and retrodiscal vasculature.

Summary

TMJ surgical decision-making rests on the disciplined integration of anatomy, imaging interpretation, and operative landmarks. MRI defines the soft-tissue phenotype that selects between arthroscopic and open intervention; CT and CBCT

Table 4 Critical distances and surgical thresholds

Structure	Distance	Surgical Relevance
Glenoid fossa roof thickness (mean)	~0.9 mm	Middle cranial fossa penetration risk during arthroscopic puncture
Middle meningeal artery to condylar apex	19 mm	Medial capsule danger zone
Middle meningeal artery to medial condylar point	15 mm	Medial capsule danger zone
Maxillary artery to sigmoid notch	6–7 mm	Risk during vertical ramus osteotomy, condylectomy
Masseteric artery to condylar neck	4 mm	Risk during arthroscopy and open exposure
Masseteric artery to articular tubercle	3 mm	Risk during eminence reduction
Masseteric artery to sigmoid notch	1 mm	Risk during osteotomy and instrumentation
Facial nerve (temporal branch) to lateral condylar pole	3–10 mm	Open approach danger zone
Facial nerve (temporal branch) crossing zygomatic arch	8–35 mm anterior to EAC	Dissect deep to superficial deep temporal fascia
Arthroscopic posterolateral portal	10 mm anterior to tragus, 2 mm inferior to tragus–canthus line[7]	Initial puncture into superior joint space
Arthroscopic anterolateral portal	20 mm anterior to tragus, 10 mm inferior to tragus–canthus line[7]	Working portal, established under visualization
Rule of 2s (capsule to neurovascular bundle)[5]	~2 cm medial to medial capsule	Working envelope for medial capsular dissection

Abbreviation: EAC, external acoustic meatus.

define the osseous corridor that determines portal trajectory, prosthesis fit, and vascular safety. Quantitative landmarks—fossa roof thickness, arterial-to-condyle distances, the Holmlund-Hellsing line, and the rule of 2s—translate this information into intraoperative execution. Future advances in dynamic MRI, 3D reconstruction, virtual surgical planning, and AI-driven analysis will continue to refine the imaging-to-surgery pipeline.

Clinics care points

The following procedure-oriented statements summarize the key decision rules and anatomic thresholds reviewed earlier:

- Obtain MRI before any planned arthroscopy or open disc surgery; interpret disc position using the intermediate zone method rather than the 12-o'clock method to avoid overdiagnosis of displacement.
- Treat joint effusion and retrodiscal signal change—not disc displacement alone—as the imaging signature of active intra-articular inflammation and the strongest indication for arthroscopic intervention.
- Match procedure to imaging phenotype: lysis/lavage for early internal derangement without disc deformity; arthroscopic repositioning when effusion plus retrodiscal inflammation is present; discectomy or alloplastic reconstruction for deformed, perforated discs with advanced degenerative joint disease.
- Confirm fossa anatomy and account for articular eminence inclination on CBCT before establishing arthroscopic portals; thin roofs or steep eminences require modified cannula trajectories to avoid middle cranial fossa penetration.
- Maintain the Holmlund-Hellsing line for arthroscopic portals (posterolateral: 10 mm anterior, 2 mm inferior to tragus; anterolateral: 20 mm anterior, 10 mm inferior).
- During the preauricular approach, dissect deep to the superficial layer of the deep temporal fascia and incise at 45° from the zygomatic root—the temporal branch of the facial nerve crosses the arch 8 to 35 mm anterior to the external acoustic meatus.
- Respect the *rule of 2s* for medial dissection (~2 cm skin-to-lateral capsule, ~2 cm lateral-to-medial capsule, ~2 cm medial capsule-to-neurovascular bundle), and obtain CT angiography in revision surgery or when anatomy appears anomalous.
- In trauma, ankylosis, and alloplastic planning, use CT (with 3D reconstruction) for condylar morphology, fossa fit, and screw-trajectory planning; in suspected condylar hyperplasia, combine SPECT/CT with CBCT for activity and morphology.
- Interpret structural imaging findings in light of the ~25% prevalence of asymptomatic abnormality—imaging confirms a clinical diagnosis, it does not establish one.

References

1. Vogl TJ, Lauer HC, Lehnert T, et al. The value of MRI in patients with temporomandibular joint dysfunction: correlation of MRI and clinical findings. Eur J Radiol 2016;85(4):714–9.

2. Tanaka E, Detamore MS, Mercuri LG. Degenerative disorders of the temporomandibular joint: etiology, diagnosis, and treatment. J Dent Res 2008;87(4):296–307.
3. Wilkes CH. Internal derangements of the temporomandibular joint. Arch Otolaryngol Head Neck Surg 1989;115:469–77.
4. Dworkin SF, Huggins KH, LeResche L, et al. Epidemiology of signs and symptoms in temporomandibular disorders: clinical signs in cases and controls. J Am Dent Assoc 1990;120(3):273–81.
5. Talebzadeh N, Rosenstein TP, Pogrel MA. Anatomy of the structures medial to the temporomandibular joint. Oral Surg Oral Med Oral Pathol Oral Radiol Endod 1999;88(6):674–8.
6. Uke WAW, Rahman FUA. Assessment of condyle head shape, fossa glenoidalis depth, and articular eminentia inclination in an adult Bugis-Makassar population. Natl J Maxillofac Surg 2025;16(2):249–55.
7. Greene MW, Hackney FL, Van Sickels JE. Arthroscopy of the temporomandibular joint: an anatomic perspective. J Oral Maxillofac Surg 1989;47(4):386–9.
8. Pullinger AG, Hollender L. Variation in condylar and fossa morphology. J Prosthet Dent 1986;55:322–30.
9. Moffett BC Jr. The morphology of the temporomandibular joint. Angle Orthod 1964;34:63–72.
10. Westesson PL. Imaging of the temporomandibular joint. Clin Radiol 1996;51:73–84.
11. Larheim TA, Abrahamsson AK, Kristensen M, et al. Temporomandibular joint imaging in adolescents. Dentomaxillofac Radiol 2015; 44:20140294.
12. Soydan D, Doğan S, Canger EM, et al. Effect of internal derangements and degenerative bone changes on the minimum thickness of the roof of the glenoid fossa in temporomandibular joint. Oral Radiol 2020;36(1):25–31.
13. Willard VP, Kalpakci KN, Reimer AJ, et al. The attachments of the temporomandibular joint disc. J Dent Res 2012;57(6):599–606.
14. Tomas X, Pomes J, Berenguer J, et al. MR imaging of temporomandibular joint dysfunction. Radiographics 2006;26(3):765–81.
15. Pereira FJ, Lundh H, Westesson PL. Microscopic changes in the retrodiscal tissues of painful TMJs with disc displacement. J Oral Maxillofac Surg 1996;54(4):461–8.
16. Farfán C, et al. Anatomical and histological components of the bilaminar zone: review. Int J Morphol 2021.
17. Emshoff R, Rudisch A, et al. Disk displacement of the temporomandibular joint: MR imaging findings. AJR Am J Roentgenol 2002.
18. Bordoni B, Varacallo M. Anatomy, head and neck, temporomandibular joint. In: StatPearls/NCBI Bookshelf, StatPearls [Internet]. Treasure Island (FL): StatPearls Publishing; 2026.
19. Vogl TJ, Günther D, Weigl P, Scholtz JE. Diagnostic value of dynamic magnetic resonance imaging of temporomandibular joint dysfunction. Eur J Radiol Open 2021;8:100390.
20. Schönegg D, Ferrari R, Ebner J, et al. Proximity of the middle meningeal artery and maxillary artery to the mandibular head and mandibular neck as revealed by three-dimensional time-of-flight magnetic resonance angiography. Oral Maxillofac Surg 2022;26(1): 139–46.
21. Rajab BM, Sarraf AA, Abubaker AO, et al. Masseteric artery: anatomic location and relationship to the temporomandibular joint area. J Oral Maxillofac Surg 2009;67(2):369–71.
22. Cuccia AM, Caradonna C, Caradonna D, et al. The arterial blood supply of the temporomandibular joint. Imaging Sci Dent 2013;43: 37–44.
23. Raposo LH. Considerations for the spread of odontogenic infections-diagnosis and treatment. In: A Textbook of Advanced Oral and Maxillofacial Surgery2. London, UK: IntechOpen; 2015. p. 341.
24. Woltmann M, Faveri RD, Sgrott EA. Anatomical distances of the facial nerve branches associated with the temporomandibular joint in adult negroes and caucasians. Braz J Morphol Sci 2000;17 (2):107–11.
25. Al-Kayat A, Bramley P. A modified pre-auricular approach to the temporomandibular joint and malar arch. Br J Oral Surg 1979;17 (2):91–103.
26. Bertram S, Rudisch A, Innerhofer K, et al. Diagnosing TMJ internal derangement and osteoarthritis with magnetic resonance imaging. J Am Dent Assoc 2001;132(6):753–61.
27. Petscavage-Thomas JM, Walker EA, et al. Advanced imaging of the temporomandibular joint. AJR Am J Roentgenol 2014.
28. Amin MF, Hassan AM, Barakat KI. The accuracy of dynamic magnetic resonance imaging in evaluation of internal derangement of the temporomandibular joint; comparison with arthroscopic findings. Egypt J Radiol Nucl Med 2012;43(3):429–36.
29. Provenzano Mde M, Chilvarquer I, Fenyo-Pereira M. How should the articular disk position be analyzed? J Oral Maxillofac Surg 2012;70 (7):1534–9.
30. Hasan NMA, Abdelrahman TEF. MRI evaluation of TMJ internal derangement: degree of anterior disc displacement correlated with other TMJ soft tissue and osseous abnormalities. Egypt J Radiol Nucl Med 2014;45(3):735–44.
31. Henderson MJ, Wastie ML, Bromige M, et al. Technetium-99m bone scintigraphy in mandibular condylar hyperplasia: false positives with TMJ disease. Clin Radiol 1990;41(6):411–4.
32. López DF, Ríos Borrás V, Muñoz JM, et al. SPECT/CT correlation in unilateral condylar hyperplasia. Diagnostics (Basel) 2021;11(3): 477.
33. del Castillo Pardo de Vera JL, Cebrián Carretero JL, Aragón Niño Í, et al. Virtual surgical planning for TMJ reconstruction with stock prostheses: pilot study. Medicina (Kaunas) 2024;60(2): 339.
34. Neuhaus MT, Zeller AN, Bartella AK, et al. Accuracy of guides/real-time navigation in TMJ replacement drilling. Dent J (Basel) 2021;9 (8):87.

Arthrocentesis and Intra-articular Injection of the Temporomandibular Joint

Gabriella Tehrany, MD, DDS [a,*], Jamie Larmie, MD, DDS [b]

KEYWORDS

• Arthrocentesis • Single-port technique • Dual-port technique • Platelet-rich plasma • Hyaluronic acid

KEY POINTS

- Arthrocentesis is a minimally invasive option for anterior disc displacement without reduction, symptomatic anterior disc displacement with reduction, early degenerative joint disease, and joint arthralgia refractory to conservative measures.
- Single-port and dual-port techniques yield comparable clinical outcomes; selection is guided by joint anatomy, surgeon experience, and therapeutic objectives.
- Adjunctive intra-articular therapies (eg, platelet-rich plasma and hyaluronic acid) may improve pain and functional recovery following arthrocentesis.
- Complications are uncommon when anatomic landmarks are respected, and lavage pressure is controlled.

Introduction: nature of the problem

Temporomandibular joint disorders (TMDs) represent a broad spectrum of conditions involving the temporomandibular joint, the muscles of mastication, and associated structures. Common intra-articular pathologies include anterior disc displacement and degenerative joint disease. TMDs affect an estimated 5% to 12% of the general population, with a higher prevalence among women between 20 to 40 years of age.[1] Patients may present with

- Joint arthralgia with associated myofascial involvement and/or headache
- Mechanical symptoms (eg, clicking, popping, intermittent locking, or crepitus)
- Functional limitations in mastication, range of motion, and speech
- Otologic symptoms (eg, otalgia, aural fullness, and tinnitus)

Chronic or refractory symptoms may contribute to psychosocial sequelae, including sleep disturbances, anxiety, and depression.

Initial management of TMDs is typically conservative. First-line interventions include oral appliances, pharmacologic therapy (eg, nonsteroidal anti-inflammatory drugs, muscle relaxants), physical therapy, and behavioral modifications.

[a] Department of Maxillofacial Surgery, Kaiser Sunset Los Angeles Medical Center, 4867 Sunset Boulevard, Los Angeles, CA 90027, USA
[b] Department of Oral and Maxillofacial Surgery, University of California Los Angeles, 10833 Le Conte Avenue, CHS 53-076, Los Angeles, CA 90095, USA
* Corresponding author.
E-mail address: gabriella.m.tehrany@kp.org

Atlas Oral Maxillofacial Surg Clin N Am 34 (2026) 201–208
1061-3315/26/Published by Elsevier Inc.
https://doi.org/10.1016/j.cxom.2026.05.004

Arthrocentesis of the temporomandibular joint aims to reduce pain and improve joint mobility through mechanical lavage and hydraulic lysis of adhesions associated with intra-articular inflammation.[1–5] First described by Nitzan in 1991 as a less-invasive alternative to arthroscopy, arthrocentesis has since evolved into a well-established intermediate intervention for patients who fail conservative therapies and do not require arthroscopic or open surgical intervention.[6]

Surgical technique

Preoperative planning

Successful temporomandibular joint arthrocentesis begins with careful patient selection and diagnostic evaluation. Ideal candidates include individuals with the following:

- Acute or subacute intra-articular arthralgia
- Anterior disc displacement without reduction
- Inflammatory arthropathies
- Early degenerative joint disease

Arthrocentesis is generally less effective in patients with end-stage degenerative joint disease (eg, advanced osseous remodeling and disc perforation), in the presence of active joint infection, or when symptoms are primary myofascial in origin.

Preoperative MRI of the temporomandibular joint (TMJ) remains the gold standard for evaluating intra-articular pathology. MRI delineates disc position and morphology, joint effusion, capsular thickening, adhesions, and retrodiscal tissue integrity. The choice of lavage technique (single-port vs dual-port) and the selection of adjunctive injectate should be guided by joint anatomy, surgeon experience, and specific therapeutic objectives (Table 1).

Abbreviations

TMDs temporomandibular joint disorders
TMJ temporomandibular joint

Table 1 Summary of clinical scenarios and recommended management strategies for temporomandibular joint arthrocentesis

Clinical Scenario	Recommended Management
Mild symptoms responsive to conservative therapy (eg, oral appliance, nonsteroidal anti-inflammatory drugs, physical therapy, behavioral modification)	Continue nonoperative management
Persistent intra-articular pain/limited opening despite appropriate conservative therapy (typically ≥3 mo)	Consider arthrocentesis
Predominantly myofascial symptoms without clear intra-articular pathology	Optimize conservative and myofascial-directed therapy before minimally invasive intervention
Active joint infection, fibrous or osseous ankylosis, suspected neoplastic pathology, or advanced degenerative joint disease with severe structural changes	Arthrocentesis generally not recommended; consider open surgical management when appropriate
Need for extensive lavage, hydraulic lysis of adhesions, or treatment of significant inflammatory burden	Dual-port arthrocentesis favored
Limited joint access, technically difficult anatomy, or primary objective of intra-articular medication delivery	Single-port arthrocentesis favored
Inflammatory arthropathy or early degenerative joint disease with persistent symptoms following lavage	Consider adjunctive intra-articular therapy (eg, corticosteroid, PRP, HA)
Recurrent symptoms or limited improvement following prior arthrocentesis	Repeat arthrocentesis or arthroscopy may be considered based on imaging findings and symptom severity
Persistent structural pathology, advanced degenerative disease, ankylosis, or failure of minimally invasive management	Consider arthroscopy or open surgical intervention

Abbreviations: HA, hyaluronic acid; PRP, platelet-rich plasma.

Preparation and patient positioning

The patient is initially placed in a supine position with the head slightly elevated. The head is rotated contralaterally to the side being treated to optimize exposure of the preauricular region. Standard antiseptic preparation and sterile draping of the operative field are performed (Figs. 1 and 2). Arthrocentesis can be performed under local anesthesia alone, local anesthesia with intravenous sedation, or general anesthesia, based on patient comfort and surgeon preference. If a nasal canula is placed during sedation, then the tubing is positioned and taped superior to the surgical field.

Local anesthesia typically involves local infiltration at the planned needle entry sites. The auriculotemporal nerve and joint capsule are anesthetized (Fig. 3). Care should be taken to prevent excessive soft tissue distortion, which may obscure anatomic landmarks and compromise accuracy.

Surgical approach

Accurate identification of surface anatomy is critical for safe and effective temporomandibular joint arthrocentesis. The canthotragal (Holmlund-Hellsing) line (Fig. 4) serves as the primary axis, extending from the lateral canthus to the midpoint of the tragus. Palpation of the preauricular region during mandibular translation can assist in confirming condylar position and joint orientation. Appropriate landmark identification and entry angle control can minimize the risk of fluid extravasation, neurovascular injury, and improve lavage efficiency.

Surgical procedure

Dual-port (dual-needle) arthrocentesis

The initial puncture is performed using a 19 to 21 gauge needle attached to a 3-mL syringe containing lactated Ringer's solution. The needle is inserted at the posterior entry point, located approximately 10 mm anterior to the tragus and 2 mm inferior to the canthotragal line, to access the superior joint space (Fig. 5). Needle is advanced anteriorly and superiorly toward the glenoid fossa. The trajectory of the needle is approximately 45° medially relative to the sagittal facial plane. The depth varies depending on the patient's tissue

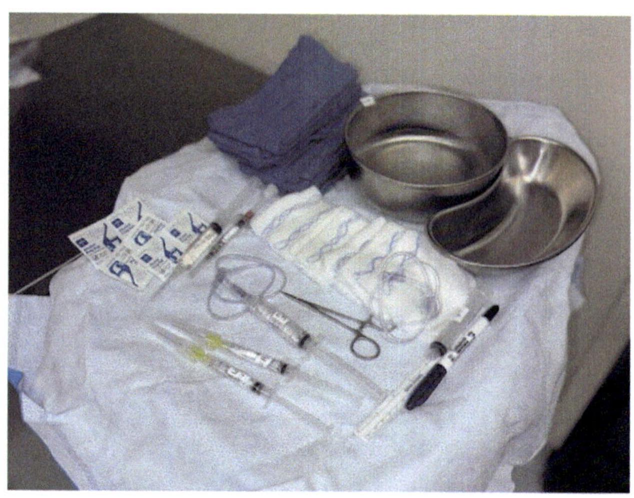

Fig. 1 Dual port procedure set up.

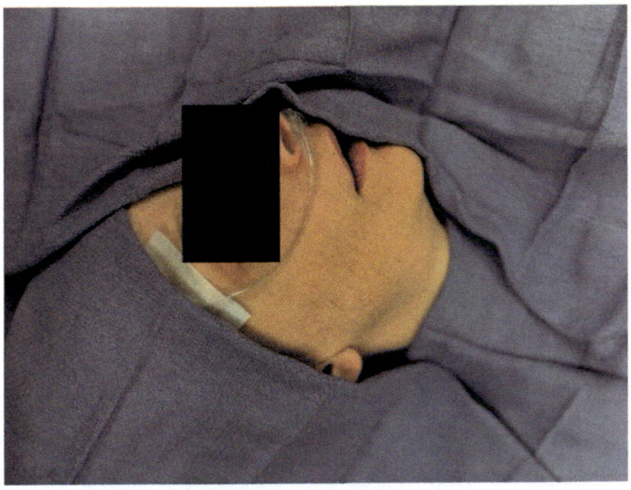

Fig. 2 Patient prep under sedation. Tape nasal canula above the field.

thickness but is typically not deeper than 20-25 mms. It is helpful to have an assistant slightly protrude and open the mandible, as the operator palpates with their nondominant hand the condylar translation during the movement. The needle is advanced slowly and gently to allow for tactile discrimination as the tip of the needle comes into contact with the temporal bone at which point the needle is slightly withdrawn and repositioned to enter more medially into the superior joint space. A sudden reduction in in tissue resistance and a subtle pop is appreciated. Correct needle placement is confirmed by aspiration of clear synovial fluid or negative pressure. A pumping maneuver, in which a small volume of fluid is injected and aspirated, producing visible fluid movement within the syringe can be observed. This maneuver should also result in observable mandibular movement (Fig. 6). Subsequently, 1 to 2 mL of solution is injected to distend the

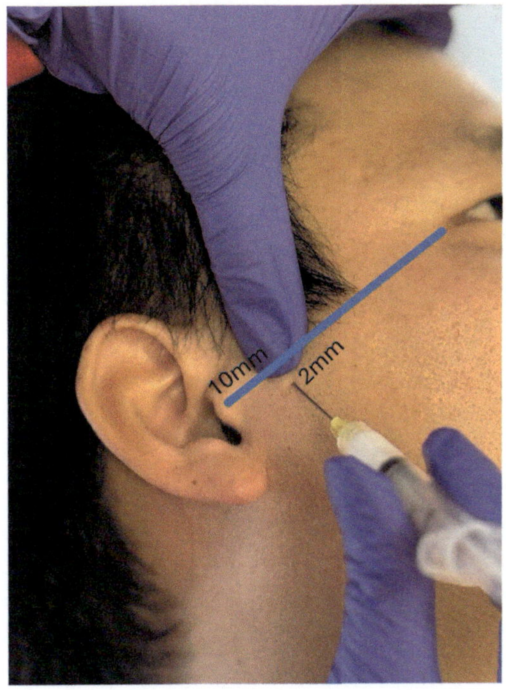

Fig. 4 Canthotragal line, single port posterior insertion.

joint space. Excessive resistance during injection may suggest extra-articular location, intracapsular fibrosis or some form of obstruction.

A second needle is then inserted at the anterior entry point, approximately 20 mm anterior to the tragus and 10 mm inferior to the canthotragal line, without attachment to a syringe (Fig. 7). The vector is directed posteriorly and slightly superomedial. The depth is slightly less—around 15 to 22 mm. Proper positioning is confirmed by spontaneous

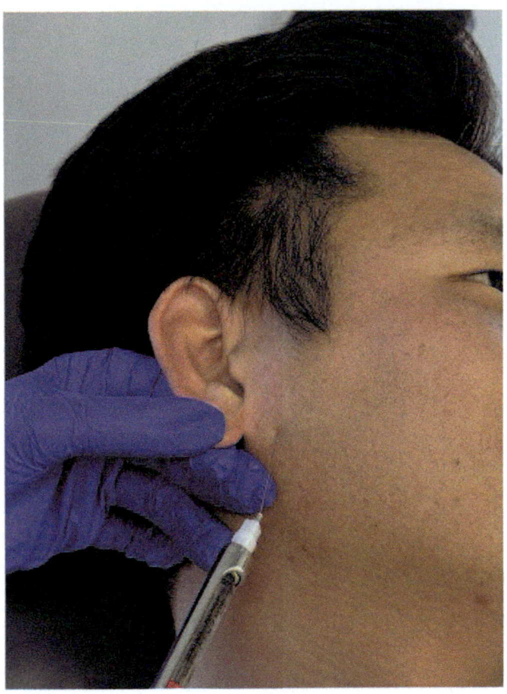

Fig. 3 Local infiltration.

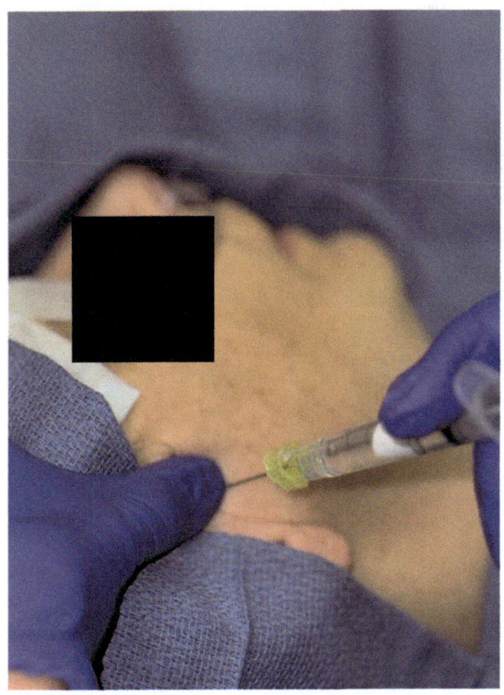

Fig. 5 Posterior point insertion.

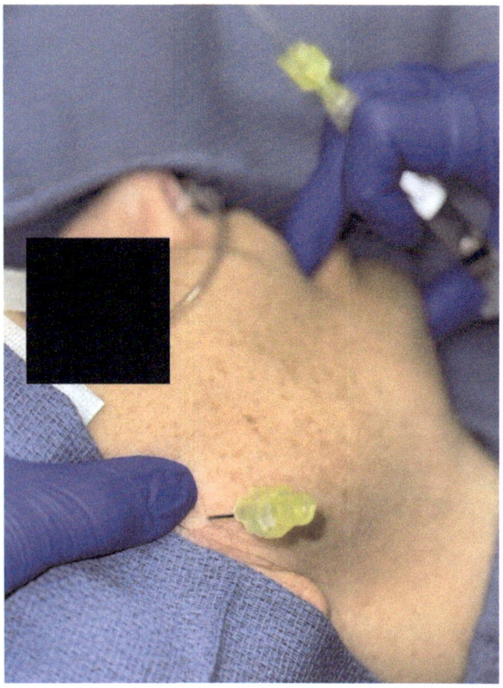

Fig. 6 Verifying placement with gentle mandible manipulation.

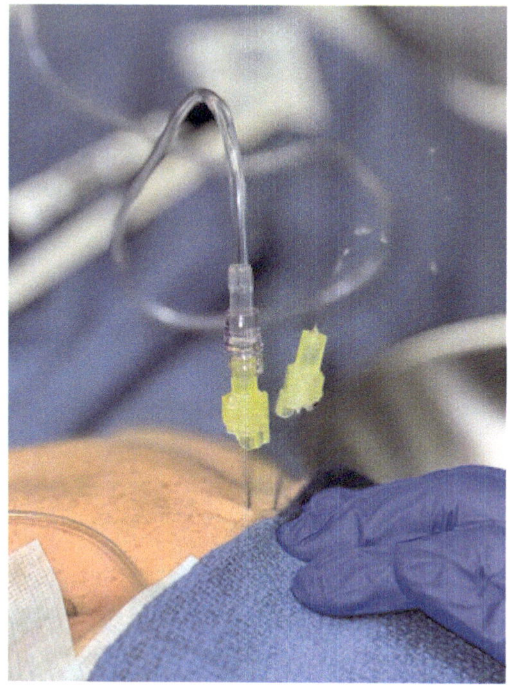

Fig. 8 Establishing flow.

efflux of fluid from the needle hub. Failure to obtain outflow should result in repositioning the needle before proceeding with irrigation. Once a bidirectional outflow has been established, extension tubing is attached, and joint lavage is performed by infusing 150 to 300 mL of solution, depending on the underlying pathology and the severity of the inflammatory disease, through the posterior needle while allowing passive drainage through the anterior needle (Figs. 8 and 9). Lavage is conducted using gentle, continuous pressure, ensuring that fluid inflow corresponds with outflow and that no extravasation into surrounding tissues occurs. Adequate lavage is characterized by low-resistance inflow and continuous outflow with absence of periarticular swelling. Initial flow may be blood-tinged and an endpoint is generally reached when outflow is visibly clearer with less particulate. An endpoint can be established not just thru the irrigation volume and appearance of the fluid, but with functional improvement observed in increased maximal opening or translation, reduction in joint resistance and smoother excursive movements.

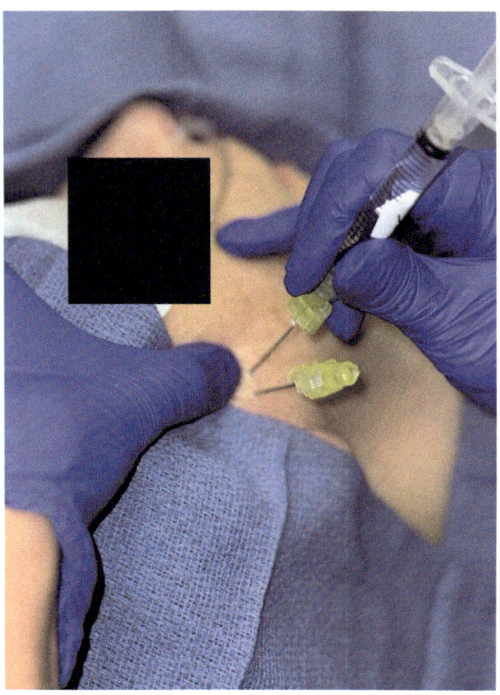

Fig. 7 Anterior port placement.

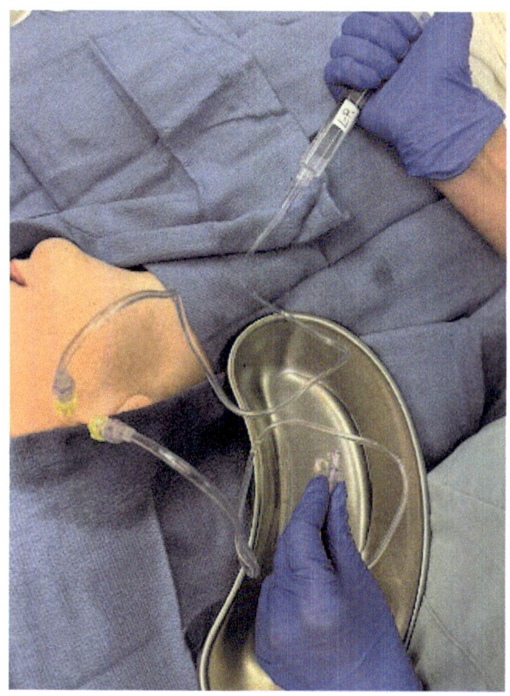

Fig. 9 Continuous lavage.

Single-port (single-needle) arthrocentesis

The single-puncture technique is an alternative approach that uses a single needle or peripheral intravenous catheter to permit inflow and outflow through one entry point (Fig. 10). A 19 to 21 gauge needle attached to a 3-mL syringe containing lactated Ringer's solution is inserted at the posterior entry point to access the superior joint space with the same vector and depth as described earlier. Correct needle placement is confirmed before initiating the procedure. Once proper positioning is established, fluid is repeatedly injected and aspirated to generate hydraulic pressure within the joint space, thereby facilitating lavage. Variations of this technique exist depending on the type of cannula employed. When a dual-lumen cannula is used, simultaneous inflow and outflow can be achieved through the same catheter. The single-puncture technique is generally less traumatic and may be technically easier to perform than dual-needle arthrocentesis. It is particularly advantageous in cases where extensive lavage is not required and the primary objective is intra-articular delivery of injectable agents, such as corticosteroids, PRP, or HA.

Intraoperative verification and trouble shooting

Failure to aspirate synovial fluid may not necessarily mean that the needle is not in the correct joint space as there is a very small amount of free fluid present. However, lack of resistance while injecting saline or extravasation of fluid may indicate extra-articular needle placement. The needle should be withdrawn slightly and repositioned. Mandibular opening with the needle in the joint space should cause it to move in congruent with the mandible if in the correct position. If there is bony contact when advancing then the needle, then withdrawal and correct repositioned done without repeated forceful advancement to minimize iatrogenic injury. Extravasation of fluid can also occur at any time after establishment of flow, if there is sudden tissue swelling, reduced outflow from the second portal or change in irrigation pressure. It is important to stop and reestablish flow by reconfirming the needle positions. Small amount of fluid leakage can occur if there are multiple punctures into the capsule and may compromise the lavage effectiveness. If there is obstruction in the flow—this may be due to synovial debris, needle bevel obstruction or improper positioning. Sometimes rotating the needle bevel or slight repositioning may help with the flow.

Adjunctive intra-articular therapies

A variety of agents have been used following arthrocentesis with the goal of improving clinical outcomes. These adjuncts include intra-articular analgesics, corticosteroids, autogenous platelet concentrates, and viscosupplementation. Among these options, corticosteroids, PRP, and HA have been the most frequently studied. These adjuncts may provide additional pain relief and functional improvement beyond arthrocentesis alone, particularly in patients with inflammatory arthropathy or early degenerative joint disease.[2,7,8]

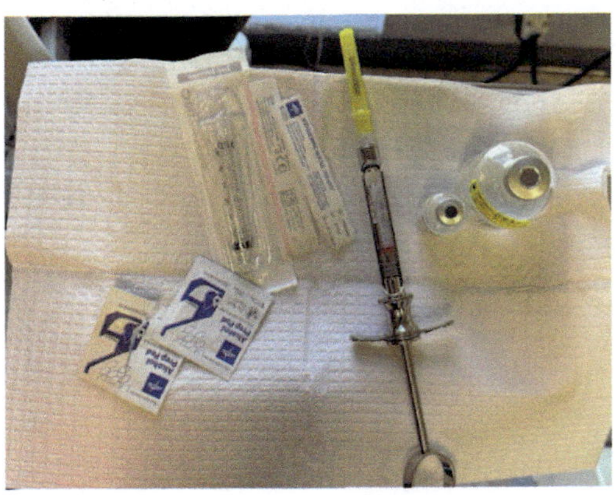

Fig. 10 Single port, no lavage set up.

Corticosteroids

Intra-articular corticosteroid injections are generally well tolerated and used for temporary relief of symptoms. A randomized, double-blind, placebo-controlled study by Dolwick and colleagues concluded that steroid supplementation following TMJ arthrocentesis results in longer-lasting pain reduction and improved pain-free mandibular mobility when compared with arthrocentesis alone. Furthermore, a systematic review evaluating arthrocentesis combined with intra-articular corticosteroids demonstrated consistent improvements in jaw function and pain relief across all included studies, with no significant adverse effects reported. However, these findings must be interpreted considering several limitations. Most studies included in the review had relatively short follow-up periods, typically ranging from 3 to 12 months.

Platelet-rich plasma

PRP is an autogenous blood derivative characterized by a supraphysiologic concentration of platelets suspended in a small volume of plasma. It belongs to a broader category of biologic agents known as autogenous platelet concentrates. These products are designed to exploit the regenerative and anti-inflammatory properties of platelets and their associated growth factors, including platelet-derived growth factor and transforming growth factor beta. The theoretic rationale of PRP as an adjunctive intra-articular injection following arthrocentesis lies in its potential to modulate inflammation and support tissue homeostasis.[9]

A small volume of PRP, usually between 1 to 2 mL, is injected intra-articularly after arthrocentesis. This sequence is intentional and allows for the following:

- Reduction of inflammatory mediators and intra-articular debris through mechanical saline lavage
- Direct interaction of PRP with synovial tissues and articular surfaces

Multiple clinical studies have reported improvements in pain scores, maximal interincisal opening, and joint function when PRP is used as an adjunct to arthrocentesis, with some suggesting longer-lasting benefits than arthrocentesis alone.[7,10,11] However, interpretation of these findings is limited due to variability in centrifugation methods, platelet concentration, leukocyte content, and injection protocols. PRP should be considered an adjunct rather than a replacement for established therapies.

Hyaluronic acid

HA is a high-molecular weight glycosaminoglycan and a major component of synovial fluid. In degenerative and inflammatory temporomandibular joint disorders, decreased endogenous HA levels and alterations in its molecular weight are associated with reduced synovial lubrication, increased intra-articular friction and progressive cartilage degradation. Intra-articular HA acts as a viscosupplement, improving lubrication and reducing inflammation.[12]

HA is typically administered in volumes ranging from 0.5 to 1.0 mL following arthrocentesis (Fig. 11). Injection protocols vary and may include a single injection or a series of injections over several weeks. When used as an adjunct therapy to arthrocentesis, multiple studies have demonstrated a greater improvement in maximal interincisal opening, pain reduction, and lateral and protrusive mandibular movements compared with arthrocentesis alone.[2,7,12] However, interpretation has been limited by variations in molecular weight, injection frequency, and study design.

HA should be regarded as an adjunctive therapy, similar to PRP. Appropriate patient selection remains critical, as HA appears to be more beneficial in degenerative and inflammatory temporomandibular joint disorders.

Potential complications

TMJ arthrocentesis has a low overall complication rate, and most adverse events are transient and self-limited. Reported complications include the following:

Fluid extravasation

Extravasation into adjacent tissues can present as preauricular fullness and discomfort. Temporary changes in occlusion related to capsular distension and periarticular swelling can occur. Risk is minimized through confirmation of intra-articular needle placement, avoidance of excessive lavage pressures, and careful control of total irrigation volume help minimize these sequelae.

Neurologic complications

Transient paresis, hypoesthesia, or paresthesia in adjacent sensory or motor nerve distributions can occur. The facial, auriculotemporal, and anterior branch of the greater auricular nerves lie near the injection site and are susceptible to injury. Proposed mechanisms include direct needle trauma, local anesthetic diffusion, and compressive effects from soft tissue edema or hematoma.

Bleeding and hematoma formation

Minor vascular injury during needle placement or lavage may result in localized swelling, ecchymosis, or hematoma in the preauricular region. These are often mild and self-limited. Risk is mitigated with careful landmark identification, attention to surface anatomy, gentle tissue handling, and avoidance of excessive lavage pressures.

Infection

Postoperative infection following TMJ arthrocentesis is rare when appropriate skin preparation and standard sterile technique is observed. Routine antibiotic prophylaxis is generally not required.

Otologic symptoms

Otologic complications are uncommon but may arise due to the proximity of the TMJ to the external auditory canal, tympanic membrane, and adjacent soft tissues. Reported manifestations include transient auricular fullness, tinnitus, vertigo, and transient Eustachian tube dysfunction. Direct injury to the middle ear cavity or external auditory canal is exceedingly rare and avoided through careful needle angulation and depth control.

Immediate postoperative care

Arthrocentesis is typically performed as an outpatient procedure. Postoperative care is focused on pain control and early

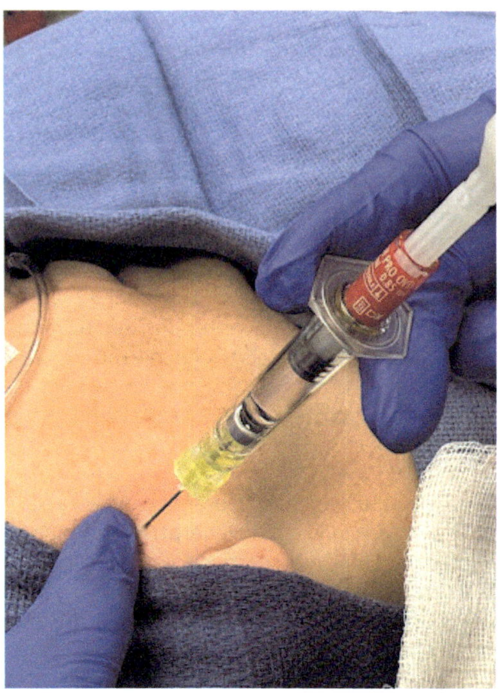

Fig. 11 Injection of HA after lavage.

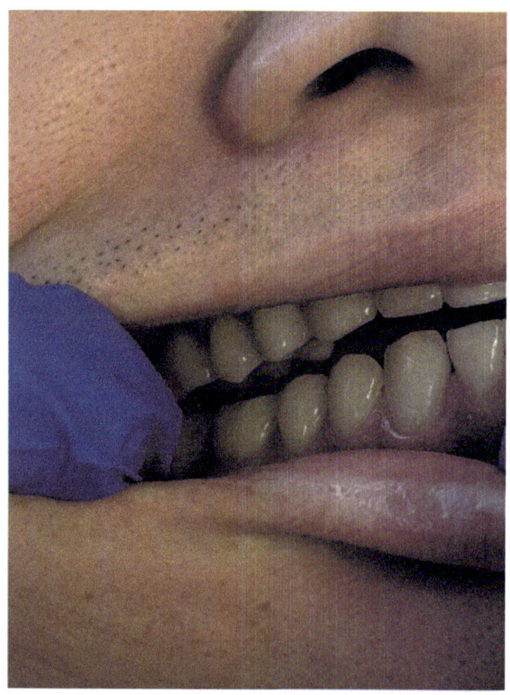

Fig. 12 Expected occlusal changes after capsule distention.

Table 2 Representative studies on temporomandibular joint arthrocentesis: techniques, outcomes, and complications

Author, Year	Sample Size	Technique	Outcomes	Complications	Follow-up Duration
Grossmann et al,[15] 2022	26	Dual-port vs single-port	Both techniques significantly reduced pain scores and increased maximal interincisal distance; no significant difference was found between techniques	No patients had complaints at final follow-up	3 y
Abbadi et al,[17] 2022	22	Arthrocentesis alone, PRP alone, or arthrocentesis combined with PRP	All groups demonstrated improvement in pain and mouth opening; greatest pain improvement was observed with arthrocentesis combined with PRP	No major complications reported	6 mo
Dolwick et al,[18] 2020; Dolwick et al,[19] 2020	24	Arthrocentesis with lactated Ringer solution followed by triamcinolone acetonide vs lactated Ringer placebo	Both groups improved after arthrocentesis; steroid supplementation provided longer-lasting masticatory-associated pain reduction at 12 wk	No major complications emphasized	6 mo

functional recovery. Nonsteroidal anti-inflammatory drugs are commonly prescribed for postoperative pain, provided no contraindications exist. A soft diet is recommended during the early postoperative period to limit joint loading and may be advanced as tolerated.

Rehabilitation and recovery

Gentle range-of-motion exercises are frequently encouraged early. Progression is guided by patient tolerance rather than a fixed protocol. Referral for physical therapy may be considered in patients with persistent myofascial pain, muscle guarding and delayed functional improvement in the absence of clear intra-articular pathology. Most patients experience improvement in pain and mobility within several weeks, with continued improvement over the following months.[13] Some patients can experience limited improvement or recurrence of symptoms after an initial response. In these situations, diagnostic reassessment is appropriate and may include repeat imaging (eg, MRI) to evaluate intra-articular pathology. Based on the clinical findings and imaging results, further management may include repeat arthrocentesis, arthroscopy, or open surgery.

Patients should be counseled preoperatively regarding the potential for transient facial nerve weakness, temporary occlusal changes (Fig. 12), postoperative edema, and sensations of increased aural pressure, all of which are typically self-limited. When doing the procedure under local, give adequate time for the anesthetic to work before inserting the needle into the joint. Let the patient know that they may feel a *swooshing* or *crunchy* sound as the fluid is moving into the joint. Occasionally the fluid going into the joint can trigger a autonomic Trigeminocardiac Reflex resulting in sudden bradycardia, hypotension and syncope. Distention of the joint can also cause Arthrokinetic Reflex and increase in electromyography activity in the jaw muscles, often felt by the patient as tightness, spasms, or increased muscle fatigue.[14]

Clinical results in the literature

Several themes are consistent throughout the literature. Outcomes (eg, pain reduction, increased maximal interincisal opening) are most predictable when symptoms are primarily intra-articular rather than myofascial in origin.[1,6] Single-port and dual-port techniques yield similar clinical results.[15] Adjunctive intra-articular therapies (eg, PRP, HA) may provide modest improvements in pain and mandibular mobility, particularly in patients with inflammatory arthralgia and early degenerative joint disease.[7,16] Interpretation of these studies are limited by variability in diagnostic group definitions, lavage parameters (eg, pressure, volume), injectate selection and dosing schedules, and duration of follow-up across studies Table 2.

Summary

Temporomandibular joint arthrocentesis is a minimally invasive option for patients with intra-articular pathology who do not respond to conservative treatment. It is commonly used to reduce pain and improve function in patients with anterior disc displacement without reduction, inflammatory arthropathy, and early degenerative joint disease. Both single-port and dual-port techniques are effective. The choice between these approaches is typically guided by joint anatomy and surgeon experience. In select patients, adjunctive intra-articular therapies, including corticosteroids, hyaluronic acid and platelet-rich plasma, may further enhance symptom relief. Complications are uncommon and generally transient when the procedure is performed with careful attention to anatomic landmarks and technique. Arthrocentesis represents a practical intermediate intervention between nonoperative care and more invasive surgical options.

Clinics care points

- *Patient Selection:* Arthrocentesis is most effective in patients with internal derangement without advanced degenerative joint disease. Contraindications include fibrous or osseous ankylosis, a history of multiple prior TMJ surgeries, active joint infection, or suspected neoplastic pathology involving the TMJ.

- *Anatomic Landmark Identification*: Accurate identification of anatomic landmarks is essential to minimize procedural complications. While the tragus-canthus line serves as a useful reference, it should not be relied upon exclusively due to individual anatomic variability. Careful palpation to identify the lateral pole of the condyle is recommended. In anesthetized patients, gentle mandibular manipulation, such as protrusion of the mandible, may assist in condylar localization. This can be performed manually by the operator or with assistance.
- *Needle Placement and Joint Access:* During needle insertion, minimizing intra-articular trauma is paramount. Multiple punctures may lead to fluid extravasation, compromise the establishment of adequate lavage flow, and increase postoperative pain and edema. If satisfactory flow cannot be achieved after multiple attempts, conversion to a single-port arthrocentesis with limited lavage followed by adjunctive intra-articular medication may be preferable to repeated attempts.
- *Intra-Articular Pressure Control:* Once flow is established, maintaining consistent and controlled intra-articular pressure is essential for effective hydraulic release of adhesions. Excessive force or high-pressure injection should be avoided, as it may increase post-operative pain or result in transient facial nerve weakness. The use of smaller syringes (10–20 mL) allows for improved pressure control. Adequate lavage volume remains necessary to facilitate the removal of inflammatory mediators.
- *Lavage Volume:* Inadequate volume of lavage may yield a suboptimum result. Although 50 milliliters of fluid can eliminate the catabolites present in the synovial fluid, if the objective is to perform adequate lavage of the joint and eliminate bradykinin, IL-6 and proteins that are inflammatory, then a larger amount (300 mL) should be used.[20] If flow is lost during this time, then occasionally repositioning the ports or changing the direction of the flow can help reestablish it.
- *Mandibular Manipulation:* Exaggerated or forceful mandibular manipulation during the procedure should be avoided to reduce the risk of capsular trauma. However, gentle mandibular mobilization and stretching following arthrocentesis may aid in adhesion release and disc mobilization, contributing to improved functional outcomes.

References

1. Liu S, Xu L, Zhang Y, et al. Do intra-articular analgesics improve outcomes after temporomandibular joint arthrocentesis? A systematic review and meta-analysis. Oral Surg Oral Med Oral Pathol Oral Radiol 2021;131(4):421–30.
2. Pérez MB, Carrasco J, Martín C, et al. Effectiveness of platelet-rich plasma in temporomandibular joint osteoarthritis: a systematic review and network meta-analysis. Int J Oral Maxillofac Surg 2025; 54(1):23–35.
3. Siewert-Gutowska M, Chęciński M, Wiśniewska G. Temporomandibular joint arthrocentesis: current concepts, techniques, and outcomes. J Craniomaxillofac Surg 2023;51(5):493–502.
4. Stout A, Friedly J, Standaert CJ. Systemic absorption and side effects of locally injected glucocorticoids. PM&R review 2019;11(4): 409–19.
5. Tang YH, Lin X, Chen Y, et al. Arthrocentesis versus conservative treatment for temporomandibular joint disorders: a systematic review and meta-analysis. Oral Surg Oral Med Oral Pathol Oral Radiol 2024;137(2):173–83.
6. Al-Moraissi EA, Wolford LM, Perez D, et al. Does arthrocentesis improve outcomes in temporomandibular joint internal derangement? A systematic review and meta-analysis of randomized controlled trials. J Oral Maxillofac Surg 2020;78(6): 944–55.
7. Kukreja P, Soni A, Mehta R, et al. Efficacy of hyaluronic acid injections in temporomandibular joint disorders: a systematic review. J Craniomaxillofac Surg 2024;52(1):12–21.
8. Li J, Liu Y, Wang L, et al. Intra-articular injection of platelet-rich plasma versus hyaluronic acid as an adjunct to temporomandibular joint arthrocentesis: a systematic review and meta-analysis. J Oral Maxillofac Surg 2024;82(7):635–46.
9. Manfredini D, Guarda-Nardini L. Arthrocentesis and minimally invasive management of temporomandibular joint disorders: an evidence-based update. Br J Oral Maxillofac Surg 2021;59(6): 643–52.
10. Nagori SA, Jose A, Roychoudhury A. Platelet-rich plasma in temporomandibular joint disorders: current evidence and future directions. Oral Maxillofac Surg Clin North Am 2023;35 (1):103–15.
11. Nemeth A, Varga G, Bender T, et al. Injectable platelet-rich fibrin as an adjunct to temporomandibular joint arthrocentesis: a systematic review. J Oral Maxillofac Surg 2024;82(10):1203–12.
12. Haddad C, Bou Serhal C, Ayoub A, et al. Platelet-rich plasma injections following temporomandibular joint arthrocentesis: a systematic review. J Stomatol Oral Maxillofac Surg 2023;124(4): 101345.
13. Bas B, Muhtarogullari M, Muhtarogullari A. The effect of exercise therapy on pain and mandibular mobility following temporomandibular joint arthrocentesis. J Oral Maxillofac Surg 2018;76(6): 1181–6.
14. Clark RK, Wyke BD. Temporomandibular arthrokinetic reflex control of the mandibular musculature. Br J Oral Surg 1975;13(2): 196–202.
15. Grossmann E, Grossmann TK, Januzzi E, et al. Single-puncture versus double-puncture arthrocentesis for disc displacement without reduction: a randomized clinical trial. J Oral Maxillofac Surg 2022;80(9):1546–54.
16. Alzahrani F, Alotaibi A, Alharbi S, et al. Arthrocentesis protocols and injectable adjuncts for temporomandibular joint disorders: a network meta-analysis of randomized controlled trials. Oral Surg Oral Med Oral Pathol Oral Radiol 2025;139(1):e1–14.
17. Abbadi W, Hattar S, Al-Qudah M, et al. Arthrocentesis alone versus arthrocentesis combined with platelet-rich plasma in temporomandibular joint osteoarthritis: a randomized controlled clinical trial. Cureus 2022;14(5):e24706.
18. Dolwick MF. Temporomandibular joint arthrocentesis: mechanisms, indications, and outcomes. Oral Maxillofac Surg Clin North Am 2020;32(1):31–44.
19. Dolwick MF, Diaz D, Freburg-Hoffmeister DL, et al. A randomized, double-blind, placebo-controlled study of the efficacy of steroid supplementation after TMJ arthrocentesis. J Oral Maxillofac Surg 2020;78:1088–99.
20. Yoshimura. The ideal lavage volume for removing bradykinin, IL-6, and protein from the TMJ. JOMS 2004;62:657–61.

Temporomandibular Joint Arthroscopy

Meshal Al Munif, DDS, SBOMFS [a], Daanesh Zakai, MBChB, BDS [b],
Mohamed Hakim, DDS, MBA [c], Clayton M. Davis, DDS, MD, MSc, FRCD(C) [a,*]

KEYWORDS

- Temporomandibular joint (TMJ) arthroscopy • Internal derangement • Chronic closed lock • Arthroscopic instrumentation
- Diagnostic and operative arthroscopy

KEY POINTS

- Temporomandibular joint (TMJ) arthroscopy is primarily indicated for intra-articular disorders, especially intra-articular pain disorder, in patients unresponsive to conservative therapy.
- Common indications include chronic closed lock, persistent pain, synovitis, adhesions, and degenerative joint disease, while contraindications include extra-articular pain and advanced ankylosis.
- Arthroscopic equipment includes small-diameter arthroscopes, cannulas, visualization systems, and specialized hand and energy-based instruments for diagnosis and treatment.
- TMJ arthroscopy is classified into 3 levels: diagnostic (level I), operative (level II), and advanced operative procedures (level III).
- A systematic 7-zone arthroscopic evaluation of the superior joint space ensures comprehensive assessment and guides surgical management.

Indications, patient selection, and decision-making

Temporomandibular joint (TMJ) arthroscopy is indicated for symptomatic intra-articular disease that persists despite appropriate conservative therapy.[1] Selection should be based on symptoms, duration, functional limitation, and imaging findings, with treatment matched to the appropriate arthroscopic level. This pathway defines when to intervene, when to escalate intraoperatively, and when open surgery or reconstruction is more appropriate. The decision process is summarized in Fig. 1.[2,3]

The main indication is intra-articular pain disorder, particularly anterior disc displacement with or without reduction, typically Wilkes stages II to IV. Arthroscopy permits lavage, lysis of adhesions, anterior release, disc mobilization, posterior scarification, and discopexy when required.[2,4–6].

Operative arthroscopy is also useful for inflammatory synovial disease of the TMJ. This includes focal or diffuse synovitis and systemic inflammatory arthropathies affecting the joint, such as juvenile idiopathic arthritis, rheumatoid arthritis, and related conditions. In these cases, arthroscopy allows lavage, synovectomy, directed biopsy when needed, and intra-articular medication delivery.

Other indications include adhesions with hypomobility, early fibrous ankylosis, disc perforation, synovial chondromatosis, painful hypermobility or recurrent dislocation, and early-to-moderate degenerative joint disease. Arthroscopy may also be diagnostic when imaging is inconclusive or biopsy is required.

Arthroscopy is not appropriate for primarily extra-articular pain, established bony ankylosis, severe joint destruction, or disease requiring open reconstruction.

Mapping clinical presentation and imaging to arthroscopic level

Clinical presentation, MRI/CT findings, and the Wilkes radiographic stage are correlated with the expected arthroscopic (Bronstein–Merrill) findings to select the procedural level (Table 1). Wilkes stages II to IV represent the principal indications; Wilkes I rarely requires arthroscopy, and Wilkes V frequently requires advanced (Level III) intervention or open surgery.[2,4,7]

Thresholds for intervention

- Failure of ≥4 to 6 weeks of structured conservative therapy (occlusal splint, physiotherapy, pharmacotherapy).[2,8]
- Closed-lock duration: acute (<1 month) and subacute (1–3 months) disc displacement without reduction respond to level I-II arthroscopy; chronic closed lock (>3 months) is preferentially treated by arthroscopy.[2]
- Persistent functional limitation, maximum interincisal opening less than 30 to 35 mm with intra-articular pain on loading.[2,9]
- Confirmed intra-articular pathology on MRI/CT, or inconclusive imaging requiring diagnostic arthroscopy.[2]

[a] Faculty of Medicine and Dentistry, University of Alberta, Canada
[b] Department of Pediatric Craniomaxillofacial Surgery, Great Ormond Street Hospital, London
[c] Department of Oral and Maxillofacial Surgery, The International Center for TMJ and Jaw Surgery, Arlington, VA, USA
* Corresponding author. Kingsway Oral Maxillofacial Surgery, 14310 111 Avenue NW, Suite 107, Edmonton, AB, T5M3Z7, Canada.
E-mail address: cmd1@ualberta.ca

Atlas Oral Maxillofacial Surg Clin N Am 34 (2026) 209-221

https://doi.org/10.1016/j.cxom.2026.05.002
oralmaxsurgeryatlas.theclinics.com

Abbreviations

RFE radiofrequency energy
TMJ temporomandibular joint

- Wilkes II to IV is the principal indication; Wilkes V often requires level III or open management.[2,7]

Contraindications

Absolute. TMJ bony ankylosis (requires open arthroplasty or joint replacement); active cutaneous, otic, or articular infection over or around the joint; and tumor with risk of intra-articular extension or seeding.[2]

Relative. Severe fibrous ankylosis or advanced osseous change (limited, often temporary benefit); severe glenoid fossa destruction or defect (risk of cranial penetration); predominantly extra-articular pain (myofascial or neuropathic); and inability to tolerate general anesthesia.[2,10]

Armamentarium

TMJ arthroscopes typically measure 1.2 to 1.9 mm in diameter and are available with 0° or 30° viewing angles.

Cannulas and trocars

Cannulas (commonly 2.0 mm in diameter) are marked in 5-mm increments to control depth. They are introduced using sharp trocars for penetration and blunt obturators for safe advancement.

Visualization systems

Arthroscopy tower: light source, HD camera, and monitors.

Basic equipment

- 22-gauge × 1.5-inch lavage needle
- French #3 myringotomy suction tip
- Intravenous tubing and stopcock
- Lactated Ringer's solution
- Local anesthetic with vasoconstrictor
- Appropriate sutures

Hand instruments

- *Probes:* straight or hooked.
- *Biopsy forceps*
- *Curette/Rasps*
- *Suction cannulas*
- *Suture-passing devices (eg, Meniscus Mender)*

Motorized and energy-based devices

- *Motorized shavers (whisker or full-radius*
- *Radiofrequency energy (RFE) (Coblation)*
- *Holmium:YAG laser*

Arthroscope selection: 0° versus 30° arthroscopes in temporomandibular joint surgery

A zero degree arthroscope provides a direct forward-facing view aligned with the instrument shaft, allowing intuitive visualization and simpler spatial orientation during TMJ arthroscopy (Fig. 2). Many modern 0° systems are *disposable arthroscopes*, offering advantages including reduced setup time, elimination of sterilization requirements, and increased accessibility. However, visualization is limited to structures directly in front of the scope, which can make the assessment of recesses and areas around anatomic contours more challenging.

In contrast, a *30° arthroscope* provides an angled field of view that allows surgeons to visualize around structures and inspect a broader area of the joint by rotating the scope. This expanded visualization is allows for comprehensive evaluation

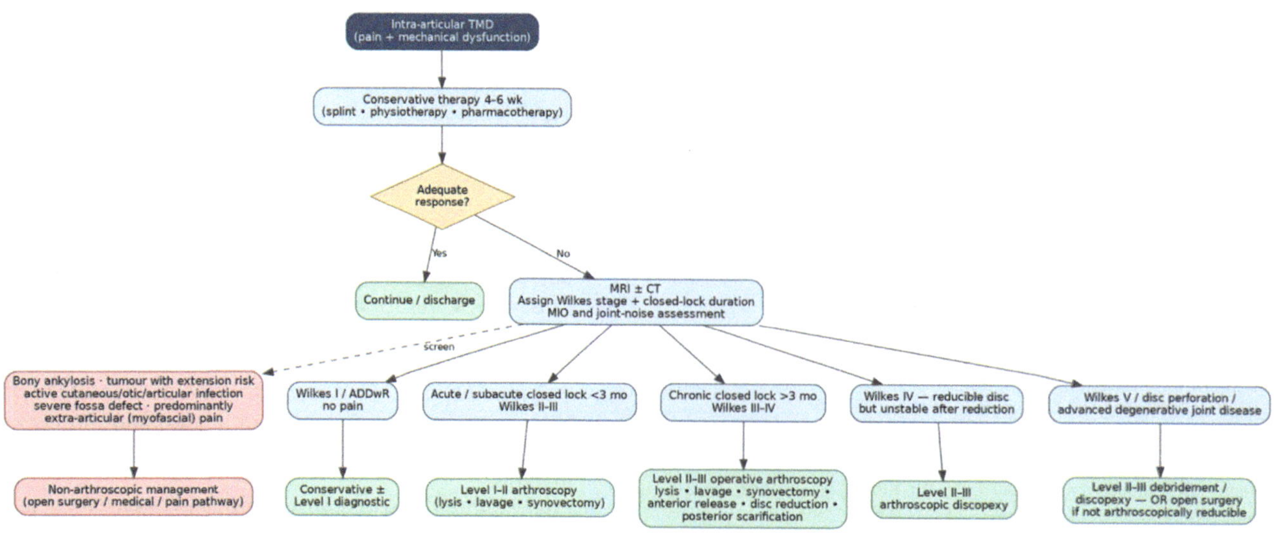

Fig. 1 Preoperative decision algorithm for TMJ arthroscopy. Clinical presentation and imaging are mapped to Wilkes stage and closed-lock duration to select the arthroscopic level; contraindications direct patients to nonarthroscopic management. ADD, anterior disc displacement; ADDwR, anterior disc displacement with reduction; DJD, degenerative joint disease; MIO, maximum interincisal opening.

Table 1 Mapping of clinical presentation, imaging (MRI/CT) findings, and Wilkes stage to arthroscopic procedural level

Clinical Presentation	Wilkes Stage	MRI/CT Findings	Arthroscopic Findings (Bronstein–Merrill)	Recommended Level
Clicking without pain; disc displacement with reduction	I	MRI: anterior disc displacement with reduction; normal disc form and marrow signal. Computed tomography (CT): normal osseous contours.	Disc *roofing* over the condyle 80%–100%; normal disc and synovium	Conservative ± Level I diagnostic
Clicking with intermittent pain; early limitation	II	MRI: disc displacement with reduction; early posterior-band thickening/mild disc deformity; ± minimal effusion. CT: normal bone.	Disc *roofing* over the condyle 50%–100%; early synovitis, anterolateral capsular prolapse, adhesions	Level I–II (lysis, lavage, synovectomy)
Acute/subacute closed lock <3 mo; ADD without reduction	II–III	MRI: anterior disc displacement without reduction; moderate disc deformity; joint effusion common. CT: normal or minimal osseous change.	Synovitis, reduced lateral recess, adhesions, chondromalacia I–II	Level I–III arthroscopy (lysis, lavage, synovectomy)
Chronic closed lock >3 mo; persistent pain/limitation	III–IV	MRI: ADD without reduction; marked disc deformity; reduced joint space. CT: early osseous change—condylar flattening, surface irregularity, small osteophytes.	Marked synovitis, adhesions, chondromalacia II–III	Level II–III (anterior release, disc reduction, posterior scarification)
ADD without reduction + early bone change; unstable after reduction	IV	MRI: ADD without reduction; hyalinized/retracted retrodiscal tissue; degenerative disc. CT: osteophytes, subchondral sclerosis, condylar and eminence flattening.	Hyalinized posterior ligament, chondromalacia III–IV	Level II–III (disc reduction + discopexy)
Crepitus; advanced DJD; disc perforation	V	MRI: disc perforation; gross disc deformity; adhesions; advanced degenerative change. CT: advanced DJD—osteophytes, erosions, subchondral cysts, sclerosis, loss of joint space.	Retrodiscal hyalinization, disc perforation, gross adhesions, chondromalacia IV	Level II–III debridement/discopexy OR open surgery
Recurrent dislocation	—	MRI: condyle anterior to the eminence crest at maximal opening; capsular laxity. CT: prominent/steep articular eminence.	Hypermobility	Level II–III eminoplasty
Hypomobility from intra-articular adhesions	—	MRI: restricted disc-condyle translation; fibrous bands; reduced recess volume/effusion. CT: usually normal osseous contours.	Fibrous adhesions, decreased recess volume	Level II lysis and lavage

Abbreviations: ADD, anterior disc displacement; CT, computed tomography; DJD, degenerative joint disease.

of intra-articular pathology. Choice of arthroscope ultimately depends on surgeon preference, experience, and procedural goals.

Classification and levels of temporomandibular joint arthroscopy

TMJ arthroscopy is conventionally divided into 3 procedural levels based on the number of ports used:

Level I: diagnostic arthroscopy

- Single-puncture technique
- Visualization of the superior joint space
- Diagnostic assessment and lavage can be considered an arthroscopy-guided arthrocentesis with the benefit of a clear understanding of the joint pathology. Arthroscopy has been shown to be superior to arthrocentesis in managing internal derangement,[11] with similar complication rates, with 4% for arthroscopy and 3% for arthrocentesis.[12]

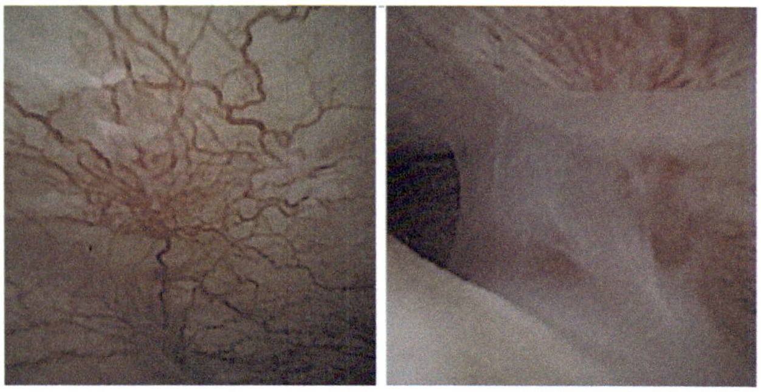

Fig. 2 Zero degree disposable scope.

Level II: operative arthroscopy

- Double-puncture technique
- Lysis of adhesions
- Lavage
- Synovectomy
- Disc manipulation
- Anterior disc release and lateral pterygoid myotomy.
- Posterior scarification

Level III: advanced operative arthroscopy

- Disc repositioning (discopexy).
- Advanced meniscal repairs
- Osteoplasty and advanced debridement with shavers
- Meniscectomy

Endoscopic anatomy of the temporomandibular joint

Arthroscopic evaluation is performed within the superior joint compartment, located between the mandibular fossa and the articular disc. A systematic examination ensures complete assessment and minimizes missed pathology.[2]

Standard 7-point arthroscopic examination

1. Medial synovial drape

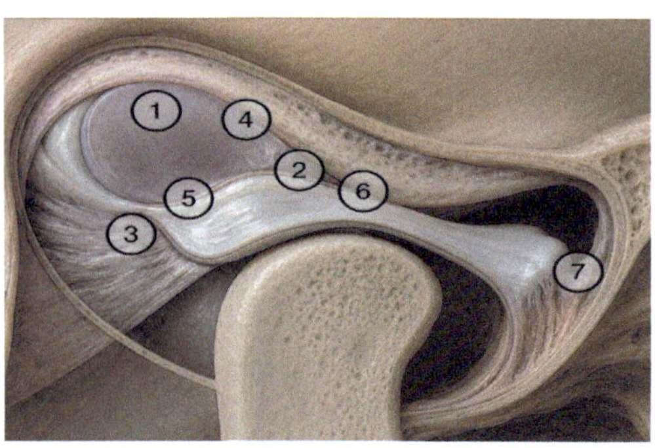

Fig. 3 The 7 points of interest of the TMJ arthroscopic examination. 1. Medial synovial drape. 2. Pterygoid shadow. 3. Retrodiskal synovium. 4. Posterior slope of the articular eminence and glenoid fossa. 5. Articular disk. 6. Intermediate zone. 7. Anterior recess.

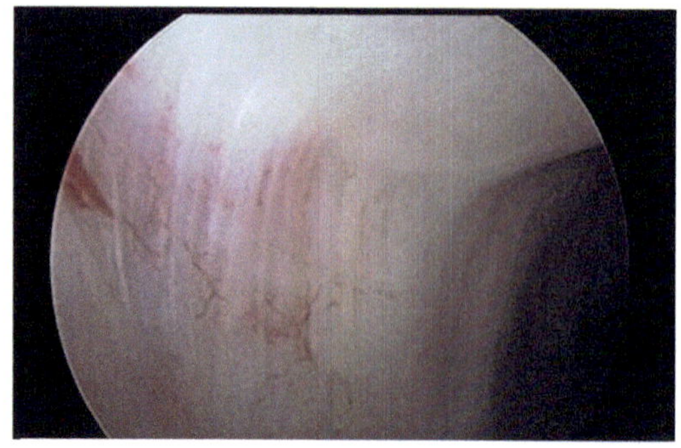

Fig. 4 Medial synovial drape.

Appears as a gray-white translucent synovial lining with vertical striations; hyperemia or fibrosis may be present (Figs. 3 and 4).

2. Pterygoid shadow
   A purplish area anterior to the medial synovium corresponding to the lateral pterygoid muscle insertion (Fig. 5).
3. Retrodiscal synovium
   Posterior attachment of the disc forming the oblique protuberance during mandibular opening (Fig. 6).
4. Posterior slope of the articular eminence and glenoid fossa
   Covered by thick fibrocartilage and commonly affected in degenerative disease (Fig. 7).
5. Articular disc
   Normally white, smooth, and avascular; assessed for mobility, perforation, or deformation (Fig. 8).
6. Intermediate zone
   Demonstrates a characteristic *white-on-white* appearance during joint motion (Fig. 9).
7. Anterior recess
   Contains the anterior synovial fold and disc-synovial crease; serves as a landmark for placement of the working portal (Fig. 10).

Surgical technique

Level I diagnostic arthroscopy (single-puncture)

Step 1: patient positioning and preparation
The procedure is performed under general anesthesia with nasal intubation. The patient is positioned supine on the operating table with the head tilted to the contralateral side and maintained in a flat position to optimize visualization of

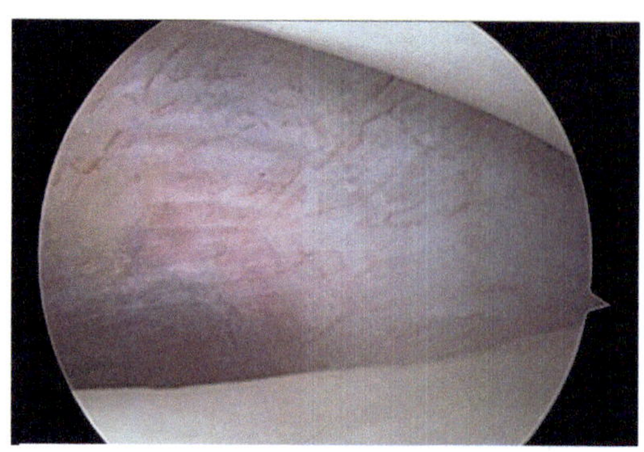

Fig. 5 Zone 2: Pterygoid shadow.

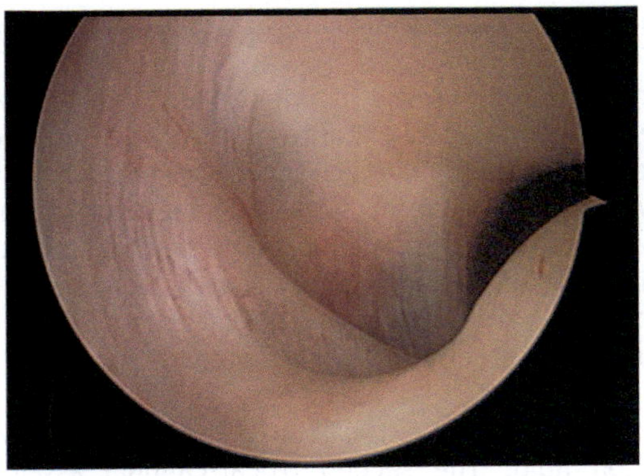

Fig. 6 Zone 3: Retrodiscal synovium.

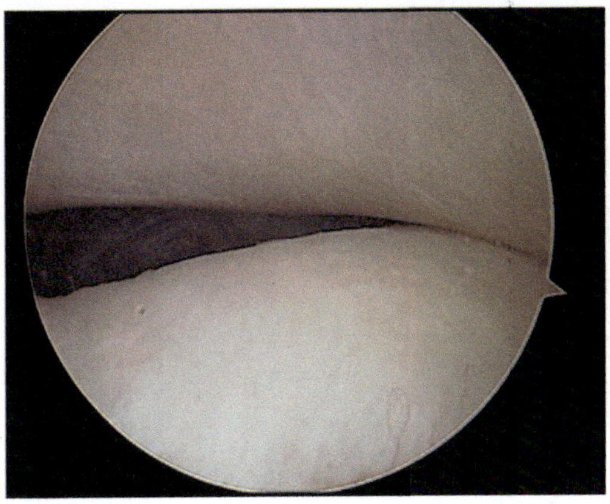

Fig. 8 Zone 5: Articular disc.

the ear and lateral canthus. Hair in the preauricular area is either shaved or held in place with silk tape.

The preauricular skin is prepared with Betadine. A sterile cotton ear pledget is placed within the external auditory canal for protection. A drape is then positioned to provide clear visualization of the ear, TMJ, and lateral canthus while allowing mandibular manipulation through the oral cavity by the surgical assistant without contamination of the operative field.[13] (Fig. 11)

The surface landmark is identified by digitally palpating the deepest concavity of the glenoid fossa (Fig. 12A–C).

Step 2: Superior joint space insufflation

Introduce a 22-gauge needle through the preauricular crease toward the glenoid fossa at approximately 45° anterior-superior angulation. Inject approximately 3 mL of saline or local anesthetic solution and confirm adequate distension by syringe plunger rebound (Fig. 13A, B).

Step 3: Fossa portal placement

The first puncture is placed at the maximum concavity of the glenoid fossa with the mandible maintained in a protruded position by the surgical assistant. The surgeon palpates the stable zygomatic process to identify the deepest point of the fossa (see Fig. 12A–C).

The trocar cannula assembly is introduced perpendicular to the skin with slight anterosuperior angulation using a slow rotational motion. The instrument is advanced until contact with the zygomatic arch is felt, typically at a depth of 5 to 10 mm (Fig. 14A–C). Maintaining bony contact, the trocar is stepped inferiorly into the superior joint space. A distinct palpable *pop* confirms capsular penetration. The cannula is advanced approximately 10 to 15 mm and should not exceed 20 to 25 mm from the skin surface, corresponding to the safety zone (Fig. 15A, B).

Step 4: Establish irrigation and visualization

The trocar is removed, and reflux of irrigation fluid confirms intra-articular placement. Continuous irrigation with lactated Ringer's solution is connected to the cannula side port (Fig. 16A, B). Insert the arthroscope into the fossa portal cannula, positioning the scope within the posterior recess (Fig. 17).

The surgical assistant insufflates the superior joint space with approximately 2 to 3 mL of lactated Ringer's solution using a direct irrigation syringe, while maintaining gentle pressure on the plunger to preserve joint distention. Under direct visualization, a 22-gauge outflow needle is inserted approximately 5 mm anterior and 5 mm inferior to the primary portal, allowing continuous irrigation throughout the procedure (Fig. 18A, B).

Step 5: First level of treatment and diagnostic arthroscopic examination

The initial stage of treatment consists of arthroscopic lavage using approximately 100 to 350 mL of irrigation fluid with turbulent flow to remove inflammatory mediators and lyse minor adhesions.

This is followed by a systematic diagnostic sweep of the superior joint space. The surgeon evaluates the 7 key zones of interest, assessing the synovium, retrodiscal tissues, articular surfaces, disc position, and joint motion. Findings such as

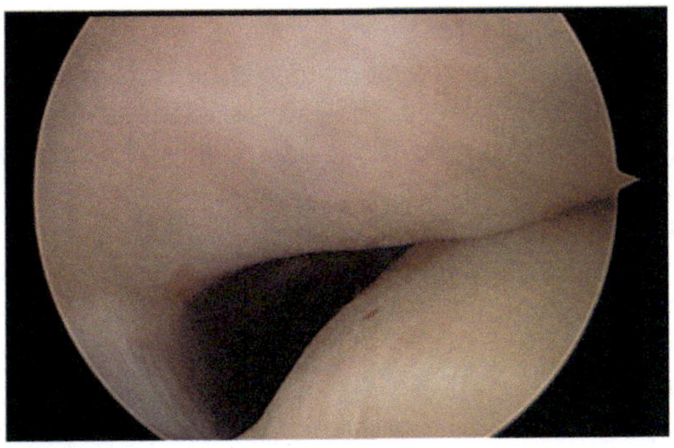

Fig. 7 Zone 4: Posterior slope of the articular eminence and glenoid fossa.

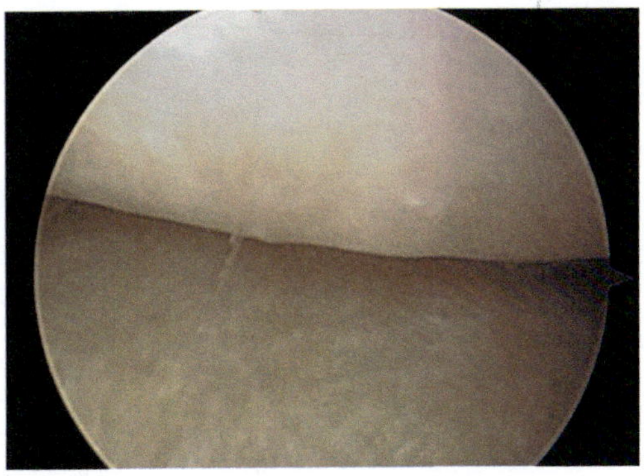

Fig. 9 Zone 6: Intermediate zone.

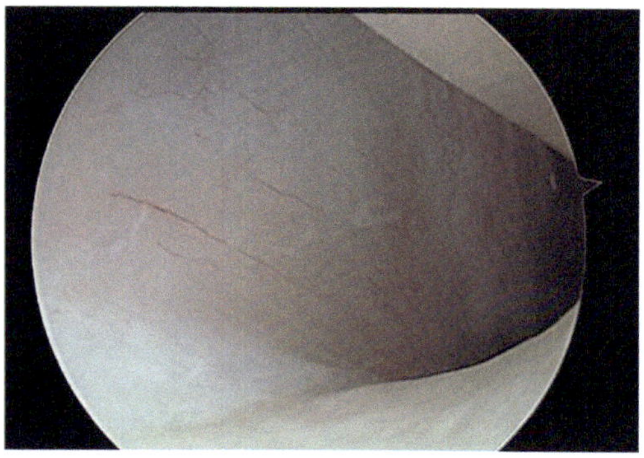

Fig. 10 Zone 7: Anterior recess.

synovitis, adhesions, fibrosis, chondromalacia, perforation, or disc displacement are documented (see Fig. 3).

If only single-puncture arthroscopy is planned, intra-articular medications may be administered at this stage as indicated, including:

- Intra-articular injection of regenerative medicine agents, including platelet-rich fibrin, platelet-rich plasma and plasma rich in growth factors, derived from the patient's own blood to promote tissue regeneration, reduce inflammation, and alleviate pain.[3,14]
- Intra-articular injection of hyaluronic acid to supplement synovial fluid, improve lubrication, and provide coverage of microbleeding surfaces.[14,15]
- Injection of corticosteroid agents into severely inflamed retrodiscal tissues

Level II operative arthroscopy (double-puncture)

Step 6: Establishment of the second puncture (working portal)

After completion of the diagnostic sweep, the arthroscope will be in the anterior recess. The condyle is seated in the glenoid fossa, the irrigation needle is removed, and the assistant depresses the mandibular molars to facilitate advancement of the scope to the most anterolateral aspect of the anterior recess (Fig. 19A, B).

The disc-synovial crease is identified, and the second puncture site is planned at this anterolateral point to maximize operative cannula mobility. Using the *vector measuring system* and *triangulation principle*, a second measuring cannula is placed flat against the skin, with its tip at the fossa portal entry site and its shaft aligned parallel to the arthroscope. The depth and direction of arthroscope penetration are transferred to the skin surface, establishing the second puncture site (Fig. 20A–C).

The assistant insufflates the joint with approximately 2 mL of irrigation fluid. The second trocar-cannula assembly is introduced perpendicular to the skin and advanced toward the junction of the anterior slope of the articular eminence and the continuation of the zygomatic arch. After bone contact, the trocar–cannula is gently redirected and rotated through the capsule and synovium into the superior joint space (Fig. 21).

Entry is confirmed under direct arthroscopic visualization. The trocar is removed, and free outflow of irrigation fluid through the cannula confirms correct intra-articular positioning. The cannula is then used as the operative working portal.

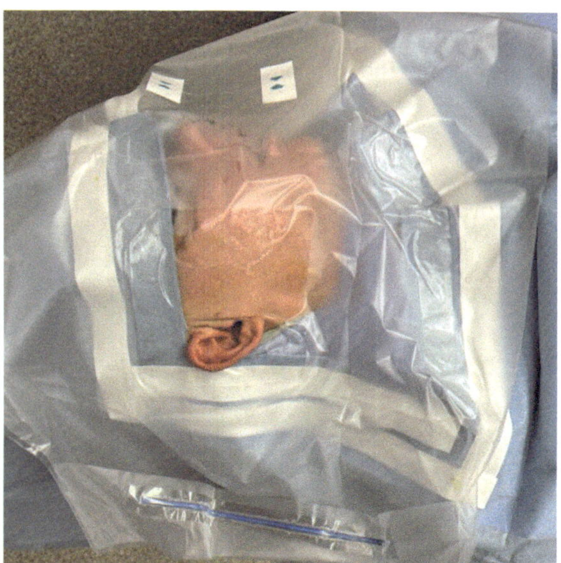

Fig. 11 Clear drape exposing the ear and preauricular area.

Step 7: Arthroscopic procedures

Lysis and lavage

A probe is used to release adhesions along the disc–synovial junction, progressing from medial to lateral compartments. Lavage restores joint volume and improves mobility.

Synovial biopsy

A full-thickness synovial biopsy is obtained using cup forceps and sent for histopathologic evaluation (Fig. 22).

Synovectomy and debridement

Hyperemic or hypertrophic synovium is ablated using radiofrequency energy (RFE/Coblation) or laser. Effective ablation is confirmed by tissue blanching.

Fibrotic tissue, adhesions, and loose intra-articular fragments are removed using probes, forceps, motorized shavers, or other instruments introduced through the second working cannula.

Debridement is performed systematically, beginning in the anterior recess, then progressing to the intermediate zone, and finally to the posterior pouch. Adequate debridement is achieved when instruments can pass freely from the anterior to the posterior joint space, with improved joint mobility and increased working space.

Anterior release

An anterior release is performed along the disc-synovial crease using coblation/RFE or laser. The release extends medially and laterally, through the synovium and capsule, to mobilize the anterior band of the disc.

The superior belly of the lateral pterygoid is partially released from its disc insertion, with the depth limited to approximately 5 mm (Fig. 23).[16]

Disc reduction

After anterior release, the arthroscope and operative cannula are moved posteriorly along the lateral sulcus toward the posterior pouch. As the instruments reach the peak of the

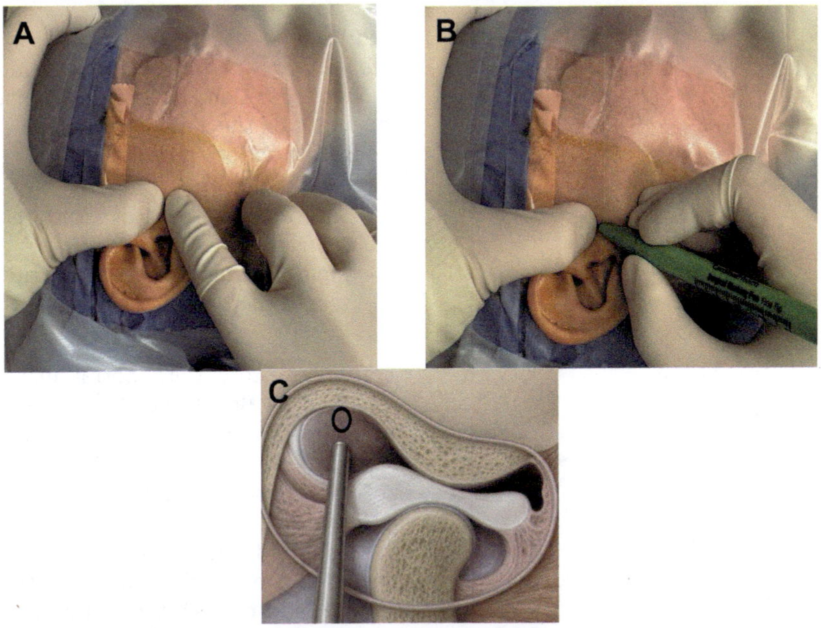

Fig. 12 (*A–C*) The fossa portal landmark is identified by digitally palpating the deepest concavity of the glenoid fossa.

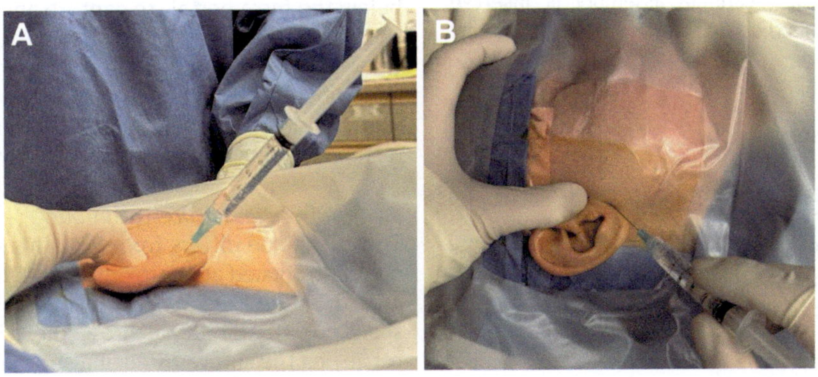

Fig. 13 (*A*, *B*) Insufflation of superior joint space by inserting a 22-gauge needle through the preauricular crease toward the glenoid fossa at approximately 45° anterior-superior angulation.

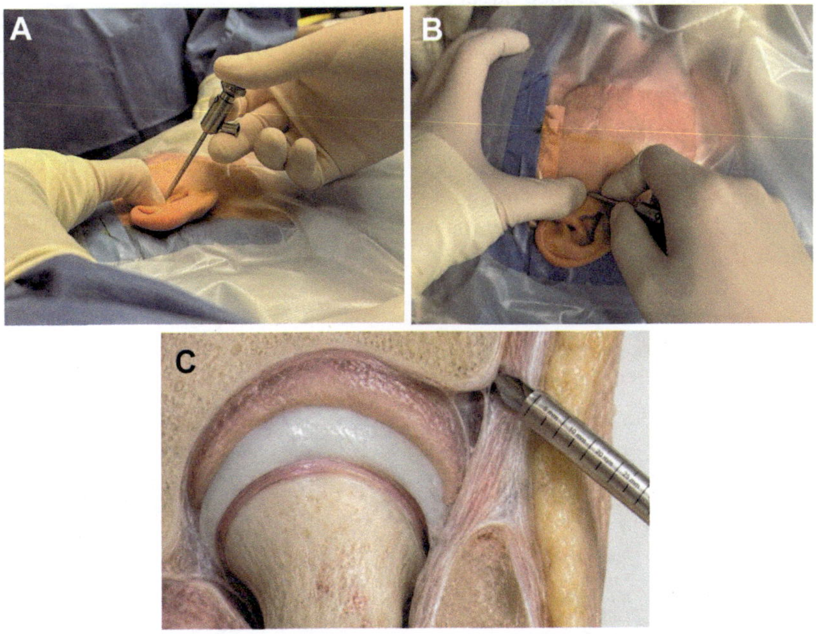

Fig. 14 (*A–C*) The trocar–cannula is inserted perpendicularly with a slight anterosuperior tilt, rotating slowly until it contacts the zygomatic arch at 5 to 10 mm depth.

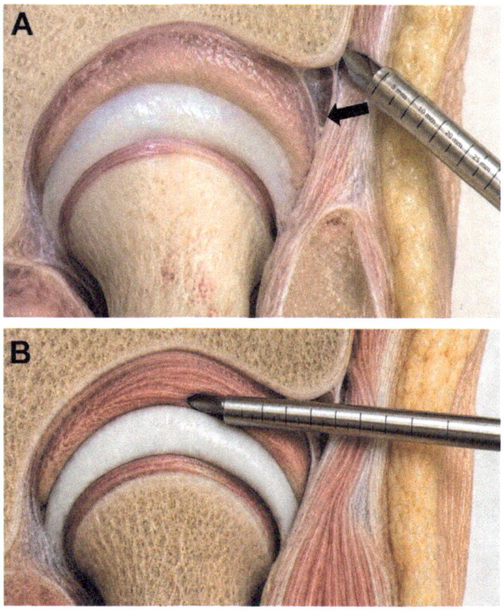

Fig. 15 (*A*, *B*) The trocar is stepped inferiorly into the superior joint space (*arrow*). The trocar–cannula assembly is inserted approximately 20 to 25 mm from the skin to the center of the joint.

articular eminence, the assistant pulls the condyle forward to facilitate entry into the posterior pouch.

The disc is reduced by applying pressure with a straight probe over the oblique protuberance of the retrodiscal tissue. Successful reduction is confirmed arthroscopically by improved disc position and increased joint mobility. Recurrent anterior displacement may still occur. Movement of the disc over the condyle helps release any inferior joint adhesions that may be present.

Posterior scarification

Controlled coblation or RFE is applied to the redundant, boggy synovium lateral to the oblique protuberance within the retrodiscal tissues posterior to the disc. Energy is applied superficially and then extended into the bilaminar zone to induce tissue contraction and improve postoperative disc stability.

Level III arthroscopy (advanced operative arthroscopy)

Level III arthroscopy includes advanced debridement, meniscectomy, disc repositioning, meniscal repair, and discopexy for Wilkes II-V internal derangement.

Arthroscopic discopexy

Disc fixation is performed after the disc is reduced and held in position. Fixation may be nonrigid, semirigid, or rigid, depending on the stability required.[13,17]

Fixation options include:

- *Suture discopexy:* 1 or 2 sutures are used to stabilize the reduced disc.
- *Rigid fixation:* resorbable or titanium screws are used to secure the disc to the condylar head.

The accessory third portal may be placed laterally, as described by McCain et al.,[13] or through a transmeatal/posterior approach to provide greater posterior traction.

McCain discopexy technique

In the McCain et al.[13] discopexy technique, the disc is reduced and stabilized arthroscopically. A 20-gauge needle carrying a Polydioxanone suture is advanced through the skin, along the condyle, and through the posterior band of the disc into the superior joint space. A straight meniscus mender is introduced through the preauricular crease, approximately 5 to 7 mm below the fossa portal, to capture and retrieve the suture. The suture is then passed from anterior to posterior and tied while the disc is held in reduction, plicating the disc to the capsule and subcutaneous tissue. Disc position, suture tension, and joint motion are confirmed arthroscopically and by manual manipulation before instrument removal.

Modified Tragal Suture technique

This technique differs from McCain's in that an 20-gauge needle is introduced at approximately 45° through the preauricular crease, and a 2-0 PDS suture is passed into the superior joint space under direct arthroscopic visualization. Instead of retrieving the suture through a second preauricular pathway, a small incision is made through the tragal cartilage within the external auditory canal. A meniscus mender with a snare is introduced through this tragal incision into the posterior pouch to capture and retrieve the suture. The suture is then passed from the tragal incision to the preauricular entry site using a Ferguson or Mayo needle and tied to plicate the disc and maintain reduction during healing (Fig. 24A–J).

Advanced arthroscopic debridement

Use motorized shavers, burrs, or coblation devices to remove advanced fibrotic tissue, loose bodies, osteophytes, or irregular condylar surfaces while preserving surrounding fibrocartilage.

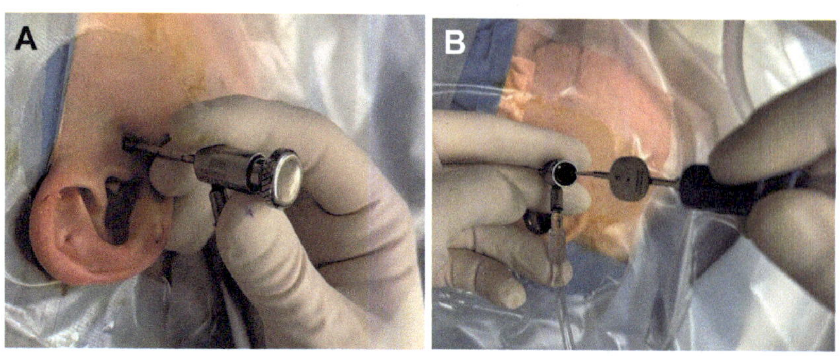

Fig. 16 (*A*, *B*) The trocar is removed, and reflux of irrigation fluid confirms intra-articular placement.

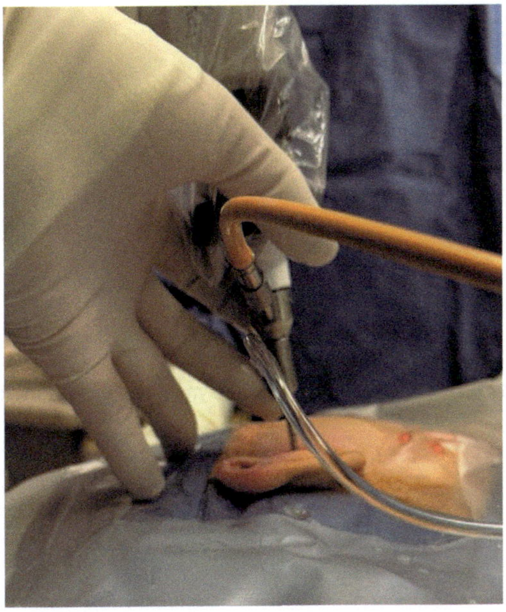

Fig. 17 The arthroscope is inserted and secured into the fossa portal cannula.

Arthroscopic eminoplasty or condyloplasty
When indicated, the articular eminence or condylar surface may be contoured using hooded burrs, motorized shavers, or other motorized instrumentation to improve joint mechanics and remove fibrotic tissue or loose fragments.

Arthroscopic eminoplasty may be performed in cases of chronic TMJ dislocation, allowing controlled reshaping of the articular eminence to reduce recurrent dislocation. This minimally invasive approach permits precise contouring while preserving surrounding soft tissues and reducing morbidity compared with open surgery.[18]

Step 8: Final arthroscopic assessment
Reinspect the joint space thoroughly and confirm hemostasis, stable disc position, unrestricted mandibular translation, and absence of instrument-related injury.

Step 9: closure
Once the procedure is complete, all instruments are removed while direct pressure is maintained over the puncture sites. The patient's head is then slightly elevated to assist with hemostasis.

The fossa puncture site is closed with a single 5-0 prolene suture, followed by application of bacitracin ointment and a small adhesive dressing. The ear pledget is then removed.

Step 10: Jaw manipulation
With the patient's head positioned upright, the surgeon manipulates and stretches the mandible, and the final range of motion is recorded.

Intraoperative decision pathways

After the systematic 7-zone diagnostic sweep, graded findings dictate the operative steps (Table 2). Operative complexity is escalated only as far as the pathology requires.[8,19,20]

Complications and management

Although TMJ arthroscopy is associated with a low overall complication rate (<4%), several complications have been reported[21]:

Neurologic

- Transient trigeminal nerve (auriculotemporal nerve) dysfunction (0.15%–2.4%)
- Temporary facial nerve (frontal branch) weakness.
- Damage can occur at the level of the central nervous system if the puncture is performed risk still exists.

Otologic

- External auditory canal laceration
- Transient hearing loss, blood clots, and lacerations of the external auditory canal were the most frequent.
- Although rare, injuries to the tympanic membrane and middle ear have been observed following arthroscopy.

Vascular

- Hemorrhage or hematoma by lesion of superficial temporal vessels, or intra-articular bleeding occurs owing to a lesion of vessels through the pterygoid muscle area, which is not usually severe and ceases after coblation of the bleeding point.
- Arteriovenous fistula (rare), treated successfully with endovascular embolization

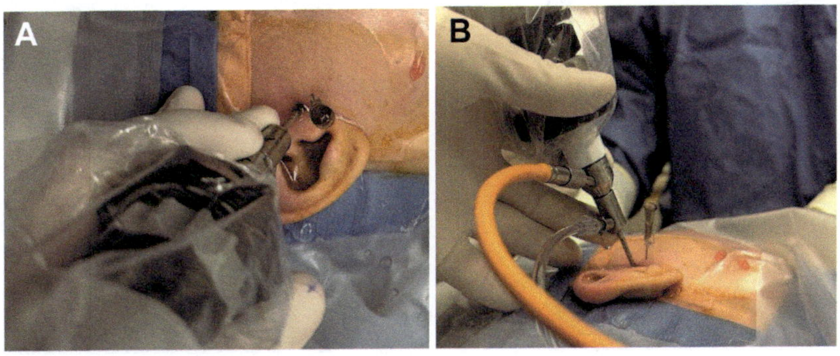

Fig. 18 (*A, B*) A 22-gauge outflow needle is inserted approximately 5 mm anterior and 5 mm inferior to the primary portal.

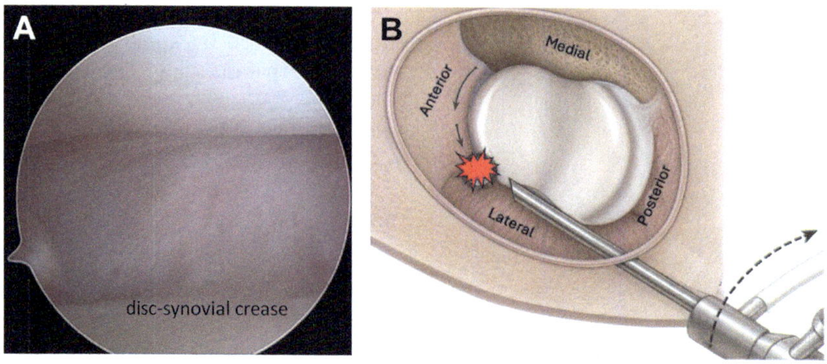

Fig. 19 (*A, B*) The arthroscope is advanced to the anteriolateral aspect of the anterior recess, and the disc-synovial crease is identified. The second puncture site is planned at this anterolateral point.

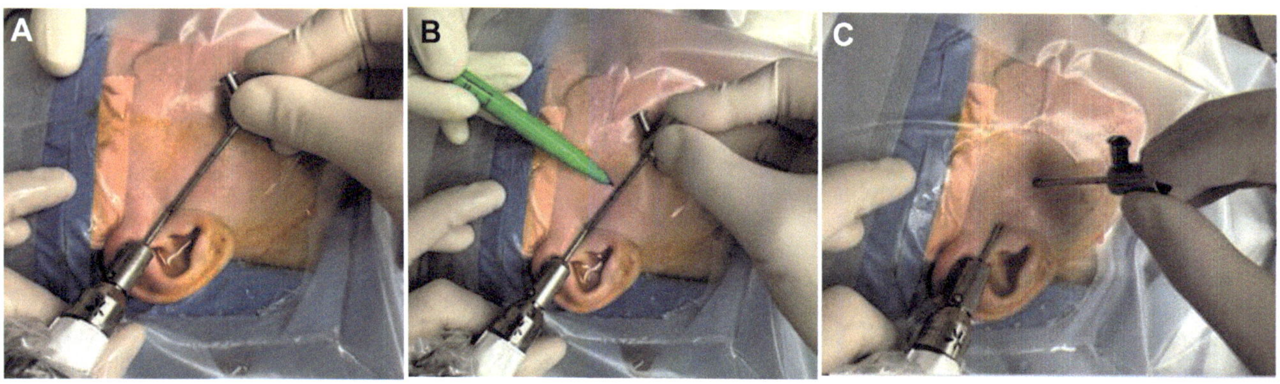

Fig. 20 (*A–C*) Double-puncture technique with vector measuring system.

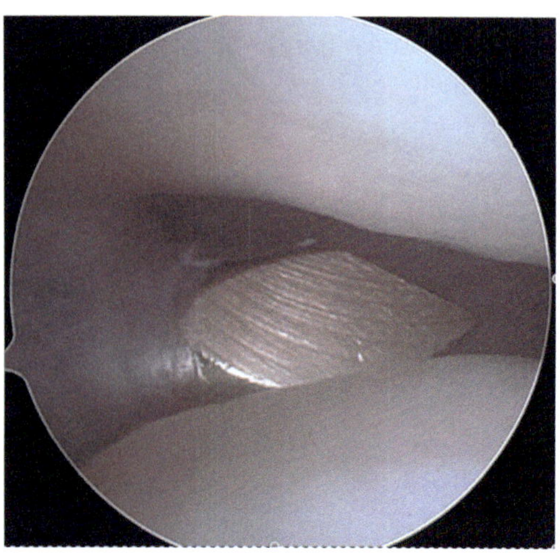

Fig. 21 Insertion of trocar-cannula assembly (second portal).

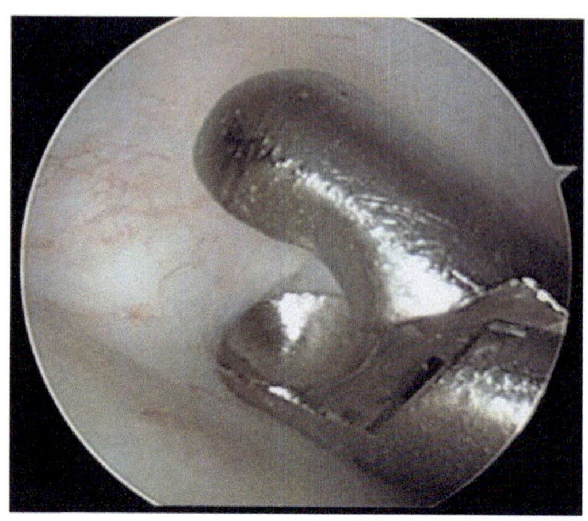

Fig. 22 Synovial biopsy.

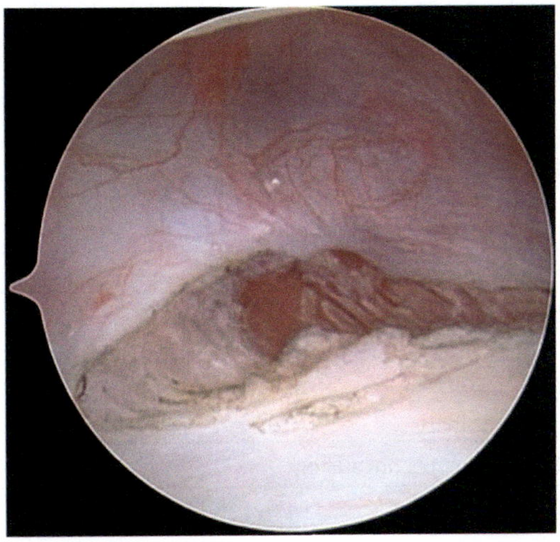

Fig. 23 Anterior release and lateral pterygoid myotomy.

Soft-tissue complications

- Facial edema due to fluid extravasation.
- Extravasation of the parapharyngeal space by irrigation fluid through an inadvertent puncture of the medial joint capsule. The patient should remain intubated until the edema resolves, typically after 24 hours.

Iatrogenic injury

- Articular cartilage scuffing during the endaural approach or discopexy.
- Instrument breakage

Postoperative malocclusion

- Which is a common occurrence in more chronic closed lock patients in which the disc is posteriorly repositioned.

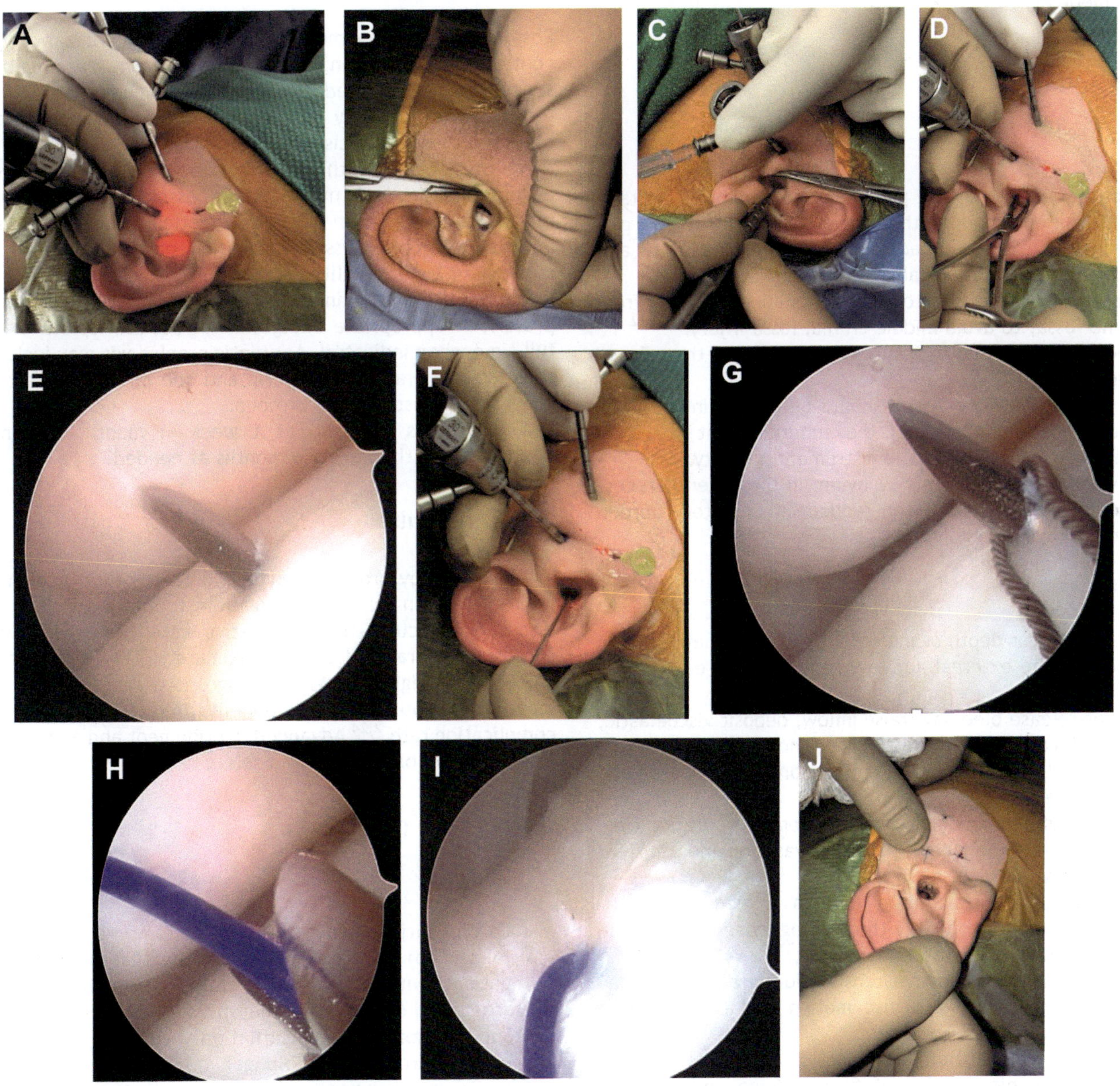

Fig. 24 (*A–J*) Modified tragal suture technique.

Table 2 Intraoperative decision pathways linking arthroscopic findings to operative actions

Arthroscopic Finding	Intraoperative Action
Synovitis (focal or diffuse hyperemia)	Coblation/Ho:YAG synovectomy until uniform blanching
Adhesions: grade 1 (silky intersynovial)	Coblation lysis
Adhesions: grade 2–3 (large anterior; disc–osseous bands)	Sharp/shaver lysis ± coblation
Reducible anterior disc displacement	Anterior release → disc reduction → posterior scarification
Disc displaced or unstable after reduction	Escalate to Level III arthroscopic discopexy
Disc perforation	Debride margins ± discopexy; large central perforation → consider open repair
Recurrent dislocation/hypermobility	Arthroscopic eminoplasty
Advanced DJD, osteophytes, irregular condyle	Condyloplasty/osseous recontouring

Abbreviation: DJD, degenerative joint disease.

Most complications are transient and resolve with conservative management.[21]

Pearls and pitfalls

Pearls

Accurately identifying the portal puncture involves digitally palpating and marking the deepest concavity of the glenoid fossa. This approach improves reproducibility and reduces the risk of portal-related complications.

Direct all instruments toward the eminence, away from the fossa, to avoid middle cranial fossa injury.[5,10,22]

Track cannula depth continuously using the 5-mm graduations.[19,22]

The second operative portal should be placed in the most anterior-lateral aspect of the superior joint space to maximize triangulation and instrument mobility.

Synovectomy of hyperemic synovium in the anterior recess and retrodiscal tissues can reduce inflammatory burden and improve pain control.

Pitfalls

Excessive trocar depth or incorrect angulation may result in injury to the external auditory canal, middle ear, or glenoid fossa.

Anterior-release bleeding: raise inflow, deposit viscoelastic, apply focal Coblation/laser, then hold 5 min external preauricular pressure with the condyle forward and contralateral.[10,19,22]

Excessive tissue manipulation and prolonged operative time increase the likelihood of fluid extravasation and transient facial nerve weakness.

Parapharyngeal extravasation through a medial capsular breach can cause airway-threatening edema; keep the patient intubated until it resolves.[10,21]

Over-reduction or excessive tension during discopexy may compromise physiologic disc motion and contribute to postoperative dysfunction.

Poor control of shavers or electrosurgical devices can produce iatrogenic scuffing of fibrocartilage and articular surface injury.

Rehabilitation and recovery

Postoperative management focuses on early mobilization, pain control, and prevention of recurrent adhesions. Patients begin supervised self-directed physiotherapy, including Stage II exercises as described by Wilk and McCain, or jaw-motion rehabilitation device exercises, typically 20 repetitions four times daily. Although mouth opening may be reduced initially because of pain, early mobilization is essential to maintain the intraoperative gain in range of motion. Therapy is later adjusted to avoid excessive translation, particularly in patients treated for hypermobility or recurrent dislocation.

Patients are maintained on a soft diet for 3 to 6 months and prescribed appropriate analgesia. An occlusal splint is worn full-time when indicated. Antibiotic prophylaxis may include a preoperative oral cephalosporin and one postoperative dose, according to institutional protocol.

Follow-up is arranged at 1 week, 1 month, 3 months, 6 months, and then every 6 months as needed.

Clinical results

TMJ arthroscopy provides reliable, durable relief of pain and improvement in mandibular function for intra-articular pain disorder refractory to conservative care. Reported overall success rates range from approximately 73% to 95% (mean ~83.5%), are highest in Wilkes stages II–IV, and improve with longer follow-up.[2,7,23] These benefits are achieved with a low complication rate.[2,24] Advanced debridement and arthroscopic discopexy can be beneficial in select cases.[5,13,25]

Clinics care points

- Careful patient selection is critical; temporomandibular joint (TMJ) arthroscopy provides the best outcomes in patients with intra-articular pathology who have failed structured conservative therapy.
- Superior joint space insufflation with local anesthetic and confirmation of plunger rebound improve safe portal establishment and facilitate arthroscopic access.

- A systematic seven-point arthroscopic examination minimizes missed pathology and improves procedural reproducibility.
- Continuous irrigation and controlled instrumentation under direct visualization minimize intra-articular bleeding, thermal injury, and iatrogenic cartilage damage.
- Limit anterior release and lateral pterygoid myotomy to a depth of approximately 5 mm, just along the disc-synovial crease, using Coblation or Ho:YAG laser.
- Disc mobility and reduction should be assessed dynamically during mandibular manipulation rather than relying solely on static arthroscopic appearance.
- Early recognition of fluid extravasation, facial swelling, or airway compromise is essential, particularly during prolonged operative arthroscopy procedures.
- Counsel chronic closed-lock patients that transient postoperative malocclusion after disc repositioning is expected and usually resolves within 2 to 8 weeks.

References

1. Badri O, Davis CM, Warburton G. Arthroscopic management and recent advancements in the treatment of temporomandibular joint disorders. Br J Oral Maxillofac Surg 2024. https://doi.org/10.1016/j.bjoms.2024.07.007.
2. González-García R. The current role and the future of minimally invasive temporomandibular joint surgery. Oral Maxillofac Surg Clin North Am 2015;27(1):27–37.
3. Gutiérrez IQ, Sábado-Bundó H, Gay-Escoda C. Intraarticular injections of platelet rich plasma and plasma rich in growth factors with arthrocentesis or arthroscopy in the treatment of temporomandibular joint disorders: a systematic review. J Stomatol Oral Maxillofac Surg 2022;123:e327–35.
4. Hossameldin RH. Usual and nonusual findings in temporomandibular joint arthroscopy. Atlas Oral Maxillofac Surg Clin North Am 2022. https://doi.org/10.1016/j.cxom.2022.06.001.
5. Askar H, Aronovich S, Christensen BJ, et al. Is arthroscopic disc repositioning equally efficacious to open disc repositioning? A systematic review. J Oral Maxillofac Surg 2021;79(10):2030–41.
6. McCain JP, Hossameldin RH. TMJ arthroscopy. In: Kademani D, Tiwana PS, editors. Atlas of oral and maxillofacial surgery. St Louis (MO): Elsevier; 2016. chap 128.
7. Bronstein SL, Merrill RG. Clinical staging for TMJ internal derangement: application to arthroscopy. J Craniomandib Disord 1992;6(1):7–16.
8. Murakami K. Rationale of arthroscopic surgery of the temporomandibular joint. J Oral Biol Craniofac Res 2013;3(3):126–34.
9. Murakami K, Segami N, Okamoto M, et al. Outcome of arthroscopic surgery for internal derangement of the temporomandibular joint: long-term results covering 10 years. J Cranomaxillofac Surg 2000; 28:264–71.
10. González-García R, Monje F. Complications of temporomandibular joint arthroscopy: a critical appraisal of the literature. J Craniomaxillofac Surg 2024. https://doi.org/10.1016/j.jcms.2024.06.018.
11. Al-Moraissi EA. Arthroscopy versus arthrocentesis in the management of internal derangement of the temporomandibular joint: a systematic review and meta-analysis. Int J Oral Maxillofac Surg 2015;44:104–12.
12. Nogueira EF, Lemos CA, Vasconcellos RJ, et al. Does arthroscopy cause more complications than arthrocentesis in patients with internal temporomandibular joint disorders? Systematic review and meta-analysis. Br J Oral Maxillofac Surg 2021;59:1166–73.
13. McCain JP, Hossameldin RH, Srouji S, et al. Arthroscopic discopexy is effective in managing temporomandibular joint internal derangement in patients with wilkes stage II and III. J Oral Maxillofac Surg 2015. https://doi.org/10.1016/j.joms.2014.09.004.
14. Fernández-Ferro M, Fernández-Sanromán J, Blanco-Carrión A, et al. Comparison of intra-articular injection of plasma rich in growth factors versus hyaluronic acid following arthroscopy in the treatment of temporomandibular dysfunction: a randomised prospective study. J Craniomaxillofac Surg 2017;45:449–54.
15. Bouloux GF, Chou J, Krishnan D, et al. Is hyaluronic acid or corticosteroid superior to lactated ringer solution in the short-term reduction of temporomandibular joint pain after arthrocentesis? Part 1. J Oral Maxillofac Surg 2017;75:52–62.
16. González-García R, Martín-Granizo R. Arthroscopic disc repositioning techniques of the temporomandibular joint. Part 1: sutures. Atlas Oral Maxillofac Surg Clin North Am 2022;30(2):175–83.
17. Zhang SY, Liu XM, Yang C, et al. New arthroscopic disc repositioning and suturing technique for treating internal derangement of the temporomandibular joint: part II–magnetic resonance imaging evaluation. J Oral Maxillofac Surg 2010;68:1813–7.
18. Cariati P, Medina BG, Galvez P, et al. Arthroscopic eminoplasty of temporomandibular joint: surgical technique. Craniomaxillofac Trauma Reconstr 2018;11(2):161–4.
19. McCain JP, editor. Principles and practice of temporomandibular joint arthroscopy. St Louis: Mosby; 1996.
20. Fernández Sanromán J, Sembronio S. Temporomandibular joint arthroscopic surgical techniques: electrocoagulation and myotomy indications. Atlas Oral Maxillofac Surg Clin North Am 2022;30(2): 165–74.
21. González-García R, Rodríguez-Campo FJ, Escorial-Hernández V, et al. Complications of temporomandibular joint arthroscopy: a retrospective analytic study of 670 arthroscopic procedures. J Oral Maxillofac Surg 2006;64(11):1587–91.
22. McCain JP, Stroia L. Arthroscopy and arthrocentesis of the temporomandibular joint. In: Miloro M, Ghali GE, Larsen PE, et al, editors. Peterson's principles of oral and maxillofacial surgery. 3rd edition. Shelton (CT): PMPH USA; 2012. p. 1069–105.
23. McCain JP, Sanders B, Koslin MG, et al. Temporomandibular joint arthroscopy: a 6-year multicenter retrospective study of 4,831 joints. J Oral Maxillofac Surg 1992;50:926–30.
24. Dimitroulis G. A review of 56 cases of chronic closed lock treated with temporomandibular joint arthroscopy. J Oral Maxillofac Surg 2002;60:519–24.
25. Ward C, Cheung J, Troost J, et al. Does postoperative disc position following double suture arthroscopic discopexy correlate with improvements in pain and quality of life. J Oral Maxillofac Surg 2025;83(5):510–27.

Open Temporomandibular Joint Surgery

Arthroplasty, Discectomy, and Disc Repositioning

Adit Gadh, DMD [a,*], Jason Adam, DDS [b,c], Joseph P. McCain, DMD [b]

KEYWORDS

• Temporomandibular joint surgery • Open arthroplasty • Discectomy • Disc repositioning • Discopexy • Arthroscopic TMJ surgery • Interpositional arthroplasty • Eminectomy

KEY POINTS

- Open temporomandibular joint surgery is indicated when advanced structural pathology exceeds the corrective capacity of arthroscopic techniques.
- Preoperative magnetic resonance imaging (MRI) and computed tomography (CT) findings must correlate with mechanical symptoms to justify surgical intervention.
- Safe dissection requires correct fascial plane identification to minimize risk of temporal branch facial nerve injury.
- Disc viability is confirmed intraoperatively under direct visualization, determining whether discopexy or discectomy is performed.
- Dynamic mandibular manipulation throughout the procedure guides operative endpoints and ensures restoration of physiologic joint translation.

Introduction

Surgical management of temporomandibular joint (TMJ) pathology has evolved toward minimally invasive and arthroscopic techniques; however, open surgery remains essential when structural disease exceeds the corrective capacity of arthroscopy—advanced internal derangement, significant degenerative change, disc perforation, dense adhesions, or failed prior procedures.[1] The objective is restoration of stable biomechanics: re-establishing the condyle–disc–fossa relationship, eliminating mechanical obstruction, and preserving condylar height. Modern TMJ surgery is a continuum; arthroscopy is the preferred approach for early and intermediate derangements, while open procedures are indispensable when advanced pathology, osseous modification, or concurrent reconstruction is required.[2,3]

Preoperative planning and patient selection

Clinical evaluation documents maximum interincisal opening (MIO), end-feel, joint sounds, occlusal stability, deviation/deflection pattern, and response to prior interventions. Progressive loss of opening, recurrent locking, or failed minimally invasive therapy indicates structural pathology. MRI evaluates disc morphology, position, mobility, perforation, and synovitis; CBCT defines osteophytes, condylar morphology, and eminence anatomy. Imaging findings are interpreted through a functional lens—they must explain the patient's mechanical symptoms to justify surgery.

Decision frameworks for approach selection (Table 1) and disc viability (Table 2) guide operative planning; final determination of disc salvageability is always confirmed intraoperatively under direct visualization.

Patient preparation and positioning

Open TMJ surgery is performed under general anesthesia with nasotracheal intubation, which preserves intraoperative occlusal assessment and jaw manipulation. Perioperative medications include prophylactic cefazolin (2 g IV within 60 minutes of incision) and dexamethasone (8–12 mg IV at induction). If the patient's cardiac status permits, administration of an anticholinergic agent (eg, glycopyrrolate) may be considered to reduce oral secretions.

The patient is placed supine with the head turned contralateral to the operative side, ensuring the zygomatic arch is parallel to the floor. The operative field includes the preauricular region, temporal scalp, and lateral orbit; the mouth is covered with a Tegaderm or Ioban to maintain a sterile field and can be accessed intraoperatively as needed. When abdominal fat harvest is planned, the periumbilical donor site is prepped concurrently.

Surgical approach and operative anatomy

Safe open TMJ surgery depends on correct plane selection. Temporal branch weakness most commonly reflects traction or

[a] Endoscopic Maxillofacial Surgery, Oral and Maxillofacial Surgery, Massachusetts General Hospital, Boston, MA, USA
[b] Oral and Maxillofacial Surgery, Massachusetts General Hospital, Boston, MA, USA
[c] Harvard School of Dental Medicine, Boston, MA, USA
* Corresponding author. Massachusetts General Hospital, Department of Oral and Maxillofacial Surgery, 55 Fruit Street, Warren 1201, Boston, MA 02114.
E-mail address: agadh@mgh.harvard.edu

Atlas Oral Maxillofacial Surg Clin N Am 34 (2026) 223-233

https://doi.org/10.1016/j.cxom.2026.05.003
oralmaxsurgeryatlas.theclinics.com

Abbreviations

MIO maximum interincisal opening
TMJ temporomandibular joint

dissection in an unsafe fascial plane rather than direct nerve injury. Three incision options are available: standard preauricular (preferred for most procedures), endaural (improved scar camouflage), and invis-incision (maximal cosmesis); a superior temporal extension is added when fascial graft harvest or extended exposure is required (Fig. 1).

Stepwise dissection and joint access:

1. Incise skin and subcutaneous tissue in the preauricular crease after epinephrine infiltration. There are 2 planes of dissection, one superior to the arch and one inferior to the arch. Superiorly, identify the superficial musculoaponeurotic system (SMAS) and superficial temporal fascia. Inferior to the arch, carry your dissection along the tragus in an avascular plane down to the capsule. Connect your superior and inferior incisions once you have identified tragal pointer at the inferior aspect of your dissection.
2. Once you identify the root of the zygoma and zygomatic arch, use Bovie electrocautery to incise down to bone. Incise periosteum over the arch and dissect subperiosteally toward the eminence, exposing the arch and lateral joint capsule. Define your superior joint space with a Freer or periosteal elevator.
3. Perform a horizontal capsulotomy at the level of the articular eminence using a Bovie or blade, entering the superior joint space. Confirm entry by direct visualization of the fibrocartilaginous articular surface.
4. Systematically inspect the superior joint space with a small retractor. Perform dynamic mandibular manipulation to localize mechanical obstruction before any instrumentation.
5. Access the inferior joint space selectively—only when disc mobilization or repositioning is planned—via the posterior attachment or separate inferior capsulotomy.

Arthroplasty

Arthroplasty eliminates mechanical interference and restores smooth condylar translation while preserving condylar height. Indications include osteophytes or irregular articular surfaces restricting translation, commonly alongside disc pathology requiring open access. Arthroplasty is a broad term that can reference alteration of the bony condyle, fossa or both. Depending on your targeted treatment, disc preserving measures should be implanted. If you are targeting the bony condyle, your intervention will take place in the inferior joint space; however if you are operating on the fossa complex, your targeted treatment will be in the superior joint space.

Table 1 Decision framework: arthroscopic versus open mporomandibular joint surgery

Favor Arthroscopic Approach	Favor Open Approach
Wilkes Stage II–IV; preserved disc morphology	Wilkes Stage IV–V; severe disc deformation or perforation
Manageable adhesions; no significant bony disease	Dense adhesions, extensive fibrosis, or prior failed arthroscopy
No concurrent osseous procedure planned	Osteophytes or eminence pathology requiring open contouring
No prior failed arthroscopic intervention	Concurrent arthroplasty, eminectomy, or graft placement planned

Table 2 Intraoperative criteria for disc salvage versus discectomy

Favor Disc Salvage (Repositioning)	Favor Discectomy
Preserved posterior band thickness (≥2 mm)	Extensive central perforation (>50% disc area)
Elastic tissue; intact fibrocartilage architecture	Diffuse thinning, fragmentation, or structural disintegration
Mobility restorable with adhesiolysis; no excessive tension	Complete loss of mobility despite thorough adhesiolysis
Absence of large central perforation	Failed prior discopexy with recurrent displacement

Final determination made under direct visualization.

1. Enter superior joint space (above the disc) and position retractors. Dynamically manipulate the mandible through full excursive range before any instrumentation—static inspection consistently underestimates functional obstruction.
2. If targeting the condyle, visualize the disc in its entirety. Place a straight hemostat along the posterior aspect of the disc, along the bilaminar zone, at the junction of the retrodiscal tissue and posterior ligaments. Use Bovie electrocautery to release the disc along the retrodiscal tissue, taking care to not violate the articular disc. The disc can now be mobilized and reflected anteriorly for access to the inferior joint space and condylar head.
3. Contour the fossa and condylar head with a small round or diamond bur (2–4 mm) under continuous irrigation. Piezoelectric devices reduce soft tissue risk when precision adjacent to capsular structures is required. Remove bone incrementally.
4. Reassess mandibular translation after each increment. Endpoint is physiologic gliding, not geometric normalization. Overresection risks irreversible occlusal change.
5. Irrigate copiously to remove bone debris. Reassess disc mobility after arthroplasty—bony correction often improves disc position and clarifies whether additional disc procedures are required.
6. Once you are satisfied with your arthroplastic maneuvers, you can reposition the disc into its native position. Use 3-0 Vicryl sutures to secure the disc back to the retrodiscal tissue and ligaments (Fig. 2).

A related but distinct indication for open joint arthroplasty arises in patients with persistent pain following total joint prosthetic reconstruction. In these cases, focal synovial entrapment, fibrous adhesions, or residual heterotopic bone around prosthetic components may produce mechanical irritation despite otherwise well-positioned hardware. Targeted

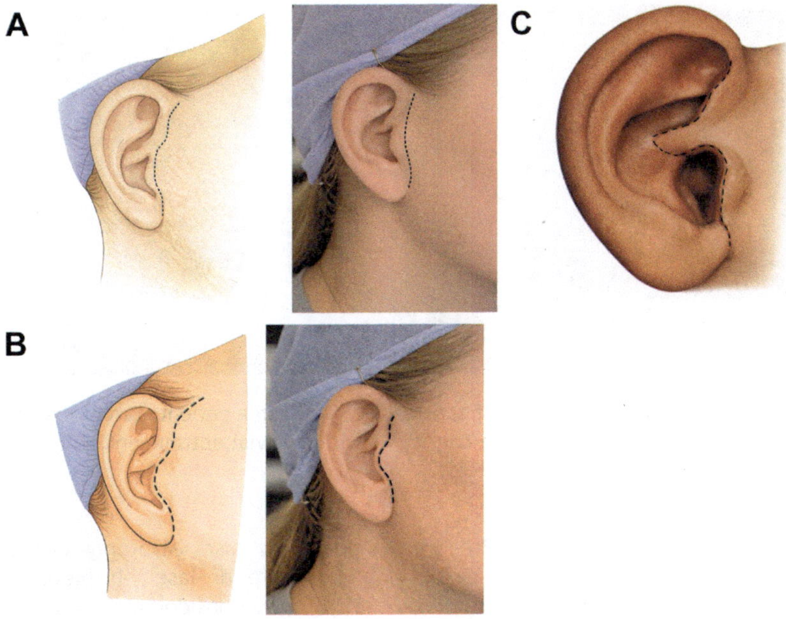

Fig. 1 (*A–C*) Incision designs for open TMJ surgery. Three representative incision patterns are shown. (*A*) The preauricular incision placed anterior to the tragus, suitable for direct access with minimal posterior extension. The incision is hidden inferiorly within a skin crease. (*B*) The endaural incision that follows the contour of the tragus and natural contours of the root of helix and lobule for improved scar camouflage. (*C*) *Invis-incision* approach that aims to virtually eliminate scar visibility.

open arthroplasty to clear restrictive tissue and restore smooth prosthetic translation can provide meaningful symptom relief without necessitating revision of the prosthesis itself (Fig. 3).

Principles of intraoperative disc assessment

Disc viability is confirmed by direct evaluation—not imaging alone. This can be done arthroscopically or under open technique. Assess posterior band thickness, surface integrity, and perforation, then evaluate disc mobility with a blunt probe. Release adhesions before judging mobility, as adhesions mimic intrinsic rigidity. Gently assess elastic recoil; a disc that collapses or buckles under minimal tension is unlikely to function after repositioning. Refer to Table 2. Tissue handling must be atraumatic; keep the field moist to minimize postoperative fibrosis.

Disc repositioning

Open disc repositioning (open discopexy)

Open discopexy is indicated for Wilkes III–IV internal derangement meeting disc salvage criteria, dense adhesions requiring open release, concomitant arthroplasty or eminectomy, or failed arthroscopic discopexy with preserved disc morphology. Anchor-based fixation with the Mitek Mini Anchor (1.8×5 mm titanium/nitinol, DePuy Synthes) is described.[4–9]

1. Enter superior and inferior joint spaces. Complete arthroplasty as indicated. Perform circumferential adhesiolysis with tenotomy scissors, releasing anterior capsular, eminence, and lateral pterygoid tethering until the disc can

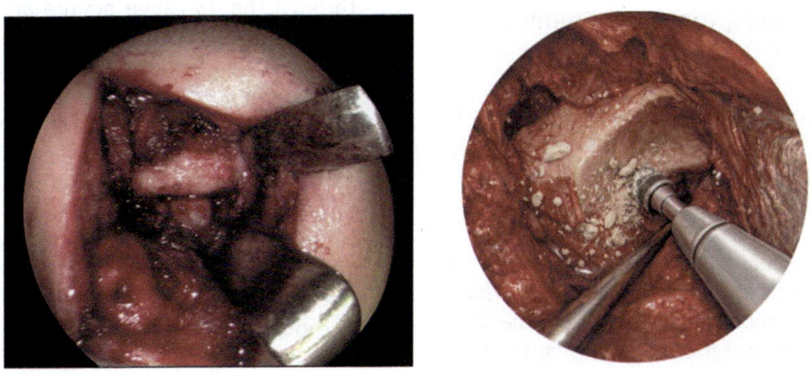

Fig. 2 Intraoperative views demonstrating inspection and conservative contouring of the superior joint space during open temporomandibular joint arthroplasty. *Left:* After capsulotomy and entry into the superior joint space, retractors expose the articular eminence and superior joint compartment for direct visualization and dynamic assessment of translation. *Right:* A small round/diamond bur under copious irrigation is used to perform incremental contouring of a focal osteophyte/irregular articular surface. Bone removal is conservative with repeated mandibular manipulation to confirm restoration of smooth physiologic translation while preserving condylar height and native joint anatomy.

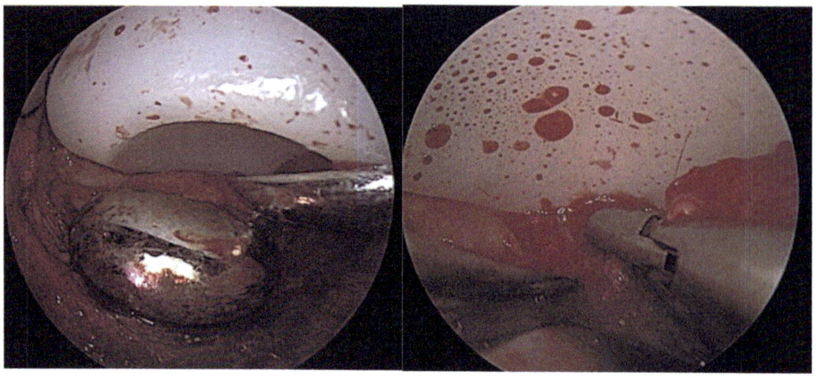

Fig. 3 Intraoperative images of a TMJ total joint replacement arthroplasty in which a patient started experiencing pain 10 years status postalloplastic joint replacement. Intraoperative findings were consistent with synovial entrapment. The synovium around the condylar head was biopsied and removed using grasping forceps and cautery.

be passively repositioned without excessive tension. Preserve the posterior attachment.

2. Hold the disc in the posterior-superior position over the condylar head with Adson forceps. Confirm natural seating without buckling. Slight overcorrection (~1–2 mm) accommodates postoperative edema.
3. Identify the anchor site: posterior-superior condylar head, 8 to 10 mm below the articular surface, just lateral to the midsagittal plane. Create a pilot hole perpendicular to the cortical surface with a 1.8 mm awl.
4. Deploy the Mitek Mini Anchor. Confirm stability by applying traction to suture tails—the anchor should not rotate or pull out under moderate traction.
5. Thread 2 2-0 Ethibond sutures through the anchor eyelet. Pass each suture through the posterior disc band in horizontal mattress configuration: one posteromedial, one posterolateral. Bites should engage adequate fibrocartilage (3–4 mm) to prevent cheese-wiring.
6. Tie sutures with the disc in the repositioned position. Tension should seat the posterior band firmly without compressing or distorting disc architecture.
7. Dynamic testing: open and close the mandible through full range. Confirm stable disc position without subluxation or restriction. Close capsulotomy with 3-0 Vicryl; layered wound closure (Fig. 4).

Arthroscopic disc repositioning (preferred minimally invasive approach)

Arthroscopic discopexy is the preferred approach at our institution for Wilkes II–IV patients with preserved disc morphology and manageable adhesions. The McCain suturing technique is described (Level III arthroscopy).[10,11]

1. Establishment of arthroscopic portals: 1st puncture is placed at the peak of the articular eminence followed by a diagnostic sweep of the superior joint space. The 2nd puncture is placed into the anterior recess using triangulation principles.
2. Disc position is assessed and the disc is mobilized using the straight probe.
3. Attention is then turned to the anterior recess, and the anterior disc crease is visualized. A pterygoid myotomy is performed along the disc synovial crease, separating the superior belly of the lateral pterygoid from the anteriorly displaced disc. Myotomy can be completed using the arthrocare or laser. If bleeding is encountered during myotomy, consider arthrocare or targeted placement of hemostatic agents (ie, Gelfoam, Surgicel). If these measures fail, withdraw your cannula systems and seat the condyle to aid in direct pressure within the joint space.
4. Once the myotomy is completed, return the operative probe to the posterior recess along the oblique protuberance. Reduce the disc into the appropriate position. When the disc is adequately mobilized, tactile feedback and direct visualization will confirm the disc *popping* back into position.
5. At this time, you can consider using the laser or arthrocare to perform contracture of the posterior ligaments.
6. The disc is now ready to be secured. Using the triangulation principle, a third portal is established with an 18-gauge needle under the reduction cannula at the level of the condylar head. It is important to understand the approximate location of the facial nerve during this maneuver, as incidence of facial nerve damage can be increased during Level III maneuvers.
7. The 18-gauge needle is walked off the condylar head, through the inferior joint space, and is visualized entering the posterior aspect of the disc.
8. A meniscus mender is placed in front of the visual cannula, and a lasso is placed through to catch the 18-gauge needle.
9. An 0-0 and 2-0 polydioxanone (PDS) suture are placed through the 18-gauge needle and secured with the lasso tool. The 18-gauge needle is removed and the lasso is withdrawn with the sutures in place. The disc can now be repositioned using the 2 sutures.
10. The 2-0 PDS suture is passed transmeatally using an eye needle and secured posterior to the tragal cartilage.
11. The 0-0 suture is secured laterally, over the skin, using a button and biopatch. Care is taken to not overtighten this suture, as it can result in skin necrosis.
12. The site is dressed and the remaining operative sites are closed with resorbable suture
13. The button and 0-0 suture are removed after 2 weeks in the clinic (Fig. 5).

Discectomy and interpositional arthroplasty

Discectomy is indicated for extensive perforation, diffuse thinning/fragmentation, severe fibrosis, or irreversible deformation. In joints with restricted access, distraction with a

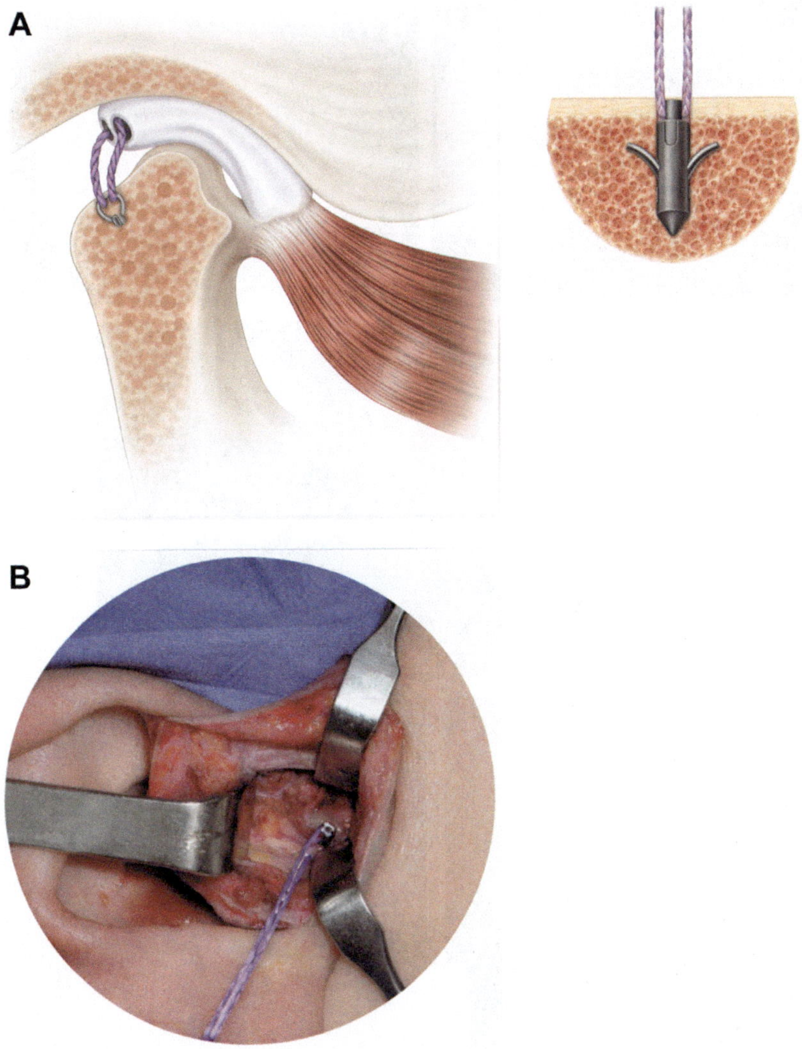

Fig. 4 (*A*, *B*) (*A*) Schematic demonstrating posterior–superior repositioning of the articular disc over the condylar head. Anchor placement to the posterior–superior condylar head with nonabsorbable sutures prepared for tension-free stabilization of the posterior band. Fixation is positioned to secure the disc without compression or distortion. Shown adjacent is a DePuy Mitek Micro/Mini Anchor (*B*) Intraoperative illustration showing open discopexy through an endaural approach. After mobilization, the disc is repositioned posterior-superiorly along the condylar head and secured with anchor-based sutures.

Wilkes retractor and K-wire or a bone-holding clamp at the mandibular angle improves visualization.[12–14]

1. Enter superior and inferior joint spaces. Begin circumferential disc mobilization laterally with Bovie electrocautery or tenotomy scissors, progressing anteromedially.
2. Remove the disc in one piece where possible. Confirm complete excision by direct visualization. Inspect condylar head and fossa surfaces; smooth irregular edges with a bur and irrigate copiously. Reassess translation dynamically—it frequently improves immediately after disc removal.
3. Achieve meticulous hemostasis of posterior joint tissues with bipolar cautery before graft placement.
4. Size and trim the interpositional graft to approximate disc dimensions (typically 2.5–3.5 × 1.5–2.5 cm). Overstuffing causes restricted opening and malocclusion; err slightly larger than the defect and assess with dynamic testing before final closure.
5. Position the graft in the superior joint space with full coverage of the fossa–condyle interface. If possible, anchor graft to the posterior capsule with 4-0 Vicryl to prevent anterior displacement. Confirm unrestricted translation dynamically.
6. Close capsulotomy with 3-0 Vicryl; layered wound closure (Fig. 6).

Graft selection is summarized in Table 3. Some joints—particularly those with smooth articular surfaces and limited degeneration—function acceptably without interposition; the decision is individualized.

Eminectomy

Eminectomy eliminates mechanical obstruction to condylar translation in recurrent dislocation or open-lock attributable to a prominent articular eminence. Selection is based on functional mechanics—not imaging alone—and is often combined with disc procedures when translational obstruction is identified intraoperatively.

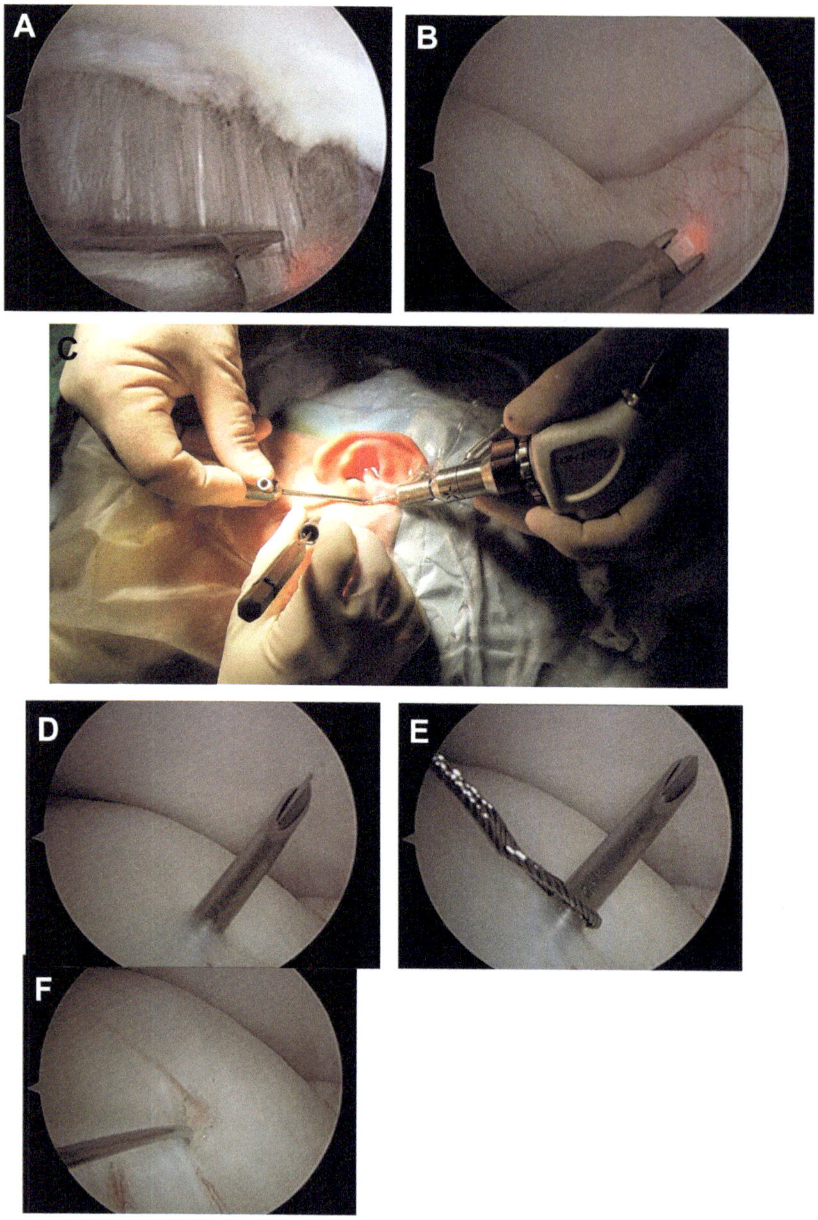

Fig. 5 *Arthroscopic Discopexy.* (*A*) Pterygoid myotomy using the laser (*B*) Posterior contracture of the retrodiscal ligaments using the laser (*C*) Establishment of third puncture using triangulation principle (*D*) Placement of an 18-gauge needle through the disc, with suture in place (*E*) Securing the 18-gauge needle with the lasso instrument (*F*) Suture in place, taut against the disc.

1. After superior joint space entry, perform dynamic mandibular manipulation to maximum opening under direct visualization. Confirm condyle–eminence mechanical obstruction at the eminence apex or anterior slope.
2. Extend subperiosteal dissection anteriorly over the full mediolateral extent of the eminence. Adequate medial exposure is essential—residual medial eminence is the most common cause of incomplete relief.
3. Begin incremental contouring at the eminence apex with a medium-large round bur (5–6 mm) or reciprocating saw; progress down the anterior slope to a level flush with or slightly below the articular fossa. Copious irrigation throughout.
4. Confirm full mediolateral completeness with a curved instrument at the medial extent. Repeat dynamic assessment after each increment—endpoint is unobstructed condylar return without forced manipulation. Avoid over-resection, which risks posteminectomy hypermobility.
5. Final smoothing with fine diamond bur. Irrigate. Close in standard layered fashion (Fig. 7).

Pearls and pitfalls

Complications and revision considerations

Temporal branch weakness is almost always neuropraxia; adherence to the subfascial plane minimizes risk and resolution is expected over weeks to months. Hematoma increases fibrosis risk; meticulous hemostasis and expanding collections require prompt management (Table 4). Transient malocclusion after disc repositioning or arthroplasty typically resolves

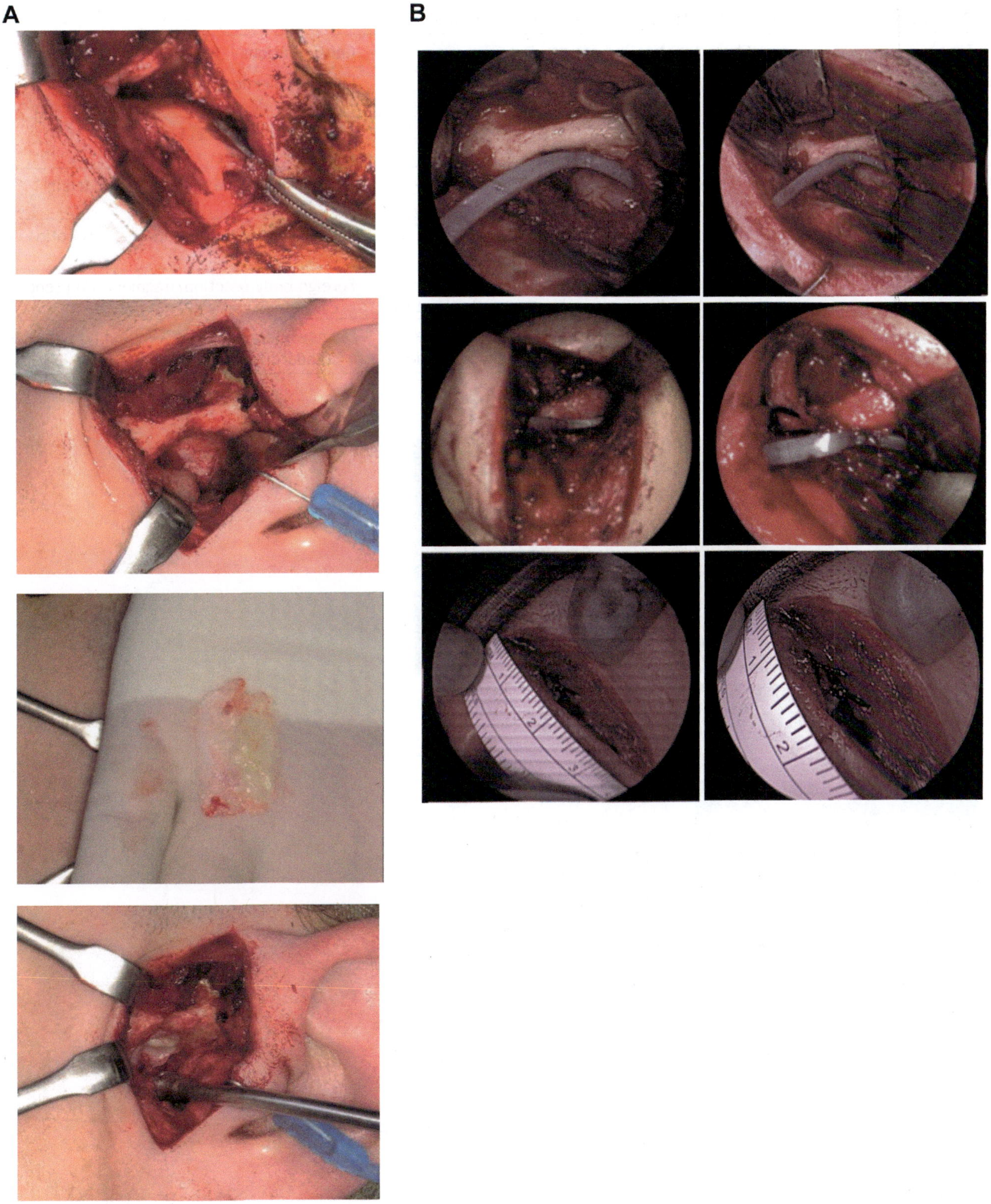

Fig. 6 (*A, B*) Sequential intraoperative images (*A*) Removal of the disc, debridement of the glenoid fossa, fabrication of a platelet-rich fibrin membrane, placement of the membrane into the superior joint space. Another interpositional option in image set (*B*), with placement of a silicone sheet and tab positioned laterally for ease of pull out. The silicone spacer is tagged to the superficial layers with a 3-0 silk suture for ease of removal at the 8 week mark. Position of the silicone tag is measured and documented. Interim placement of the silicone sheet allows for fibrous pseudo disc formation.

within 2 to 4 weeks with early mobilization; persistent occlusal change warrants assessment for condylar height loss or graft overstuffing. Limited opening most commonly reflects fibrosis from inadequate rehabilitation; arthroscopic lysis is preferred over repeat open surgery when adhesions are suspected.

Procedure-specific concerns include recurrent disc displacement (anchor pullout, tissue degeneration, or bony

Table 3 Interpositional graft selection after temporomandibular joint discectomy

Graft Type	Characteristics/Indications	Considerations
Temporalis fascia (autogenous)	Local; low morbidity; same incision. First-line autogenous option.	Limited thickness; may be insufficient in severely degenerated or revision joints
Abdominal fat (autogenous)	Biologically active; resists contraction; preferred when fibrosis risk is high.	Requires periumbilical harvest; volume loss over time
Acellular dermis (allograft)	Consistent thickness; no donor site. Useful when autogenous options are limited.	Allogenic material; variable remodeling profile
Auricular cartilage (autogenous)	Structural cartilaginous matrix; more rigid interposition option.	Donor site morbidity; potential absorption over time
Silicone spacer (alloplastic)	Temporary spacer in selected revision cases; "pull-out" technique at ~8 wk. Historical use.	Foreign body reaction/fragmentation reported; careful patient selection required
Autogenous platelet matrix/membrane	Autogenous membrane with platelet derived growth factors and regenerative properties	Unknown loading properties and no published standardized protocol

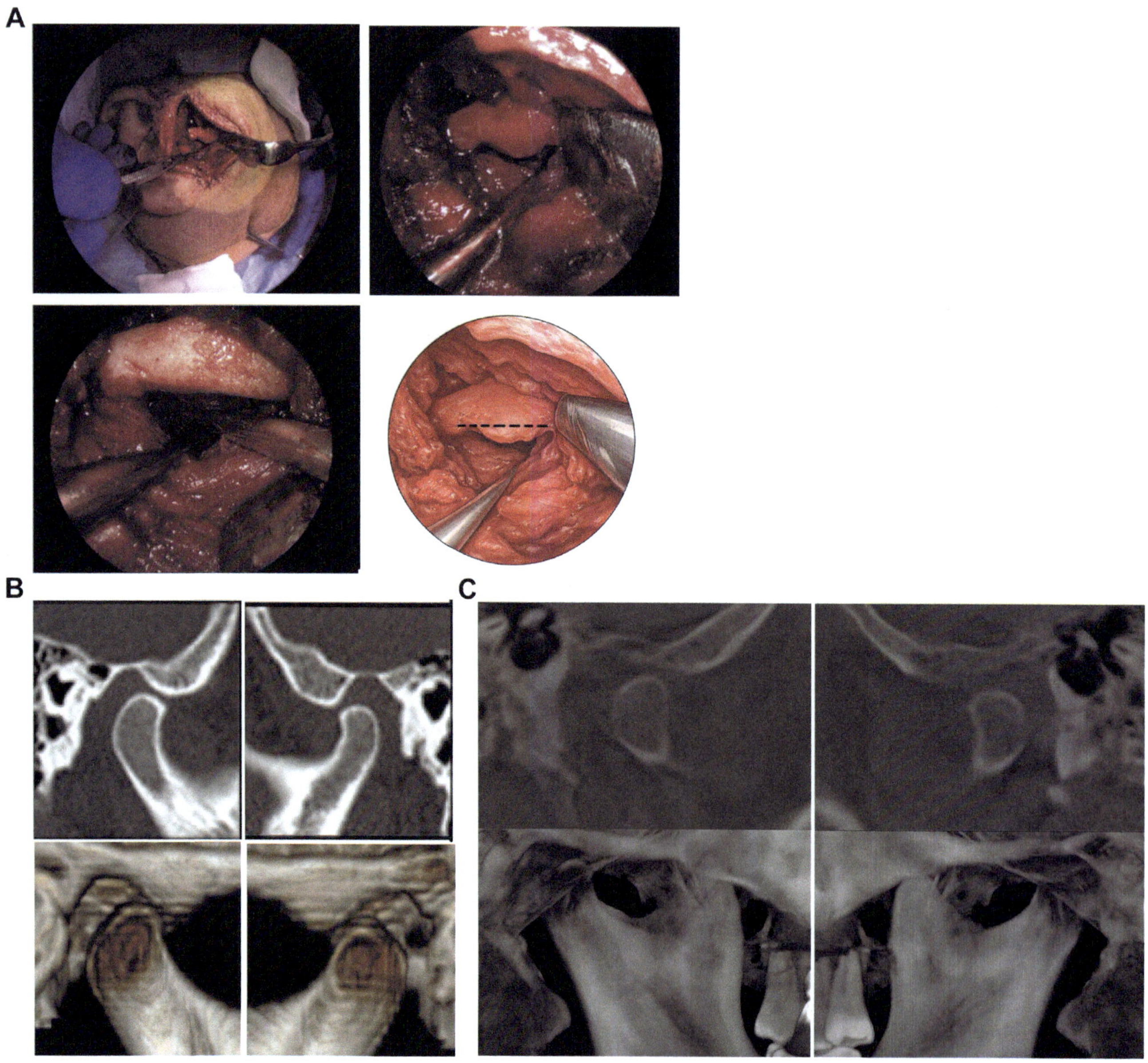

Fig. 7 (*A–C*) Composite illustration demonstrating clinical, intraoperative, and radiographic correlation in eminectomy performed for recurrent dislocation or open-lock associated with a prominent articular eminence. (*A*) Intraoperative views of contouring of the articular eminence apex and anterior slope. (*B, C*) Preoperative and postoperative imaging demonstrating radiographic flattening of the articular eminence following eminectomy.

Table 4 Pearls and pitfalls for open temporomandibular joint surgical procedures

Procedure/Step	Pearl	Pitfall to Avoid
Approach	Subfascial dissection over the zygomatic arch is the single most reliable maneuver for temporal branch protection—confirm the plane before advancing.	Avoid dissecting in the subcutaneous plane over the arch where the temporal branch is most vulnerable.
Arthroplasty	Always perform dynamic mandibular manipulation before bone removal to localize impingement precisely; static inspection consistently underestimates obstruction.	Avoid radiograph-guided resection without intraoperative functional correlation; over-resection of the condylar head is irreversible.
Disc Assessment	Release adhesions before assessing disc mobility—adhesions mimic intrinsic disc rigidity and cause premature discectomy decisions.	Do not declare a disc nonviable until adhesiolysis is complete.
Open Discopexy (Mitek)	Anchor placement 8–10 mm below the articular surface at the posterior-superior condylar head. Slight disc overcorrection (~1–2 mm) at tying accommodates postoperative edema.	Avoid anchoring too superiorly (articular surface violation) or too anteriorly (suture vector pulls disc forward).
Arthroscopic Discopexy	Confirm transdisc needle passage arthroscopically before withdrawing—suture through retrodiscal tissue only will not provide durable repositioning.	Do not apply extracapsular tension until arthroscopic confirmation of correct disc-body placement.
Discectomy	Release lateral attachment first and posterior attachment last to maintain disc position during dissection and prevent uncontrolled tearing.	Avoid posterior attachment avulsion before lateral/anterior releases—risks retrodiscal vessel injury and field obscuration.
Interposition	Size graft to match excised disc; dynamic testing before final closure is mandatory.	Overstuffing causes restricted opening and malocclusion; trim conservatively when uncertain.
Eminectomy	Address the full mediolateral extent—medial residual eminence is the most common cause of incomplete relief.	Do not assess adequacy from lateral exposure alone; palpate medial extent with a curved instrument.
Closure	Repair the capsule without overtightening—adequate translation must be preserved to prevent early adhesion formation.	Overclosure restricts translation and mimics early mechanical failure.

drivers), interpositional graft contracture or displacement, and posteminectomy hypermobility when contouring is excessive. Historical silicone implant failure—fragmentation and foreign body synovitis—requires removal with conversion to biological interposition or alloplastic reconstruction. Revision surgery should be undertaken only after objective correlation of symptoms with mechanical pathology and failure of appropriate rehabilitation; options range from arthroscopic lysis to repeat open surgery to total joint reconstruction.

Postoperative care and rehabilitation

Immediate management includes compression dressing for 24 to 48 hours, head elevation, cold therapy, and multimodal analgesia (scheduled non-steroidal anti-inlamattory drugs [NSAIDs], acetaminophen, short-course opioid rescue). Mobilization begins on postoperative day 1 with gentle, repetitive opening within a comfortable range—consistency is the goal, not maximal opening. Passive stretching devices are introduced

Table 5 Summary of published clinical outcomes

Procedure	Follow-up	Pain Improvement	Functional Outcomes	Reference
Arthroscopic discopexy (Wilkes II–III)	12 mo	86.7% primary success (pain-free at 12 mo)	Significant MIO and excursion improvement; superior outcomes Stage II–III vs IV–V	McCain et al,[10] 2015
Open discopexy (Mitek anchor)	1–4 y	75%–85% satisfactory pain outcomes	MIO improvement 5–10 mm; disc position maintained on MRI in 70%–80%	Mehra et al,[4] 2001; Marlière et al,[5] 2003
Discectomy (±interposition)	5–20 y	75%–90% long-term pain relief	MIO maintained/improved in majority; fat/fascial graft reduces fibrosis recurrence	Holmlund et al,[12] 1993; Eriksson et al,[13] 1985
Arthroplasty (functional)	1–3 y	70%–85% pain/mechanical symptom improvement	Improved MIO and excursive range; outcomes optimized with concomitant disc management	Spallaccia et al,[15–19] 2025
Eminectomy	1–2 y	Recurrent dislocation resolved >90%	Normal/near-normal translation; hypermobility rate <5% with conservative contouring	Kerstens et al,[20] 1989; Sidebottom et al,[3] 2024

selectively in high-risk patients after the peak inflammatory phase (days 3–5). After open discopexy, avoid extreme opening (>30 mm) for the first 2 weeks to protect suture and anchor integrity during early healing.

Soft diet is maintained through 6 weeks. Rehabilitation progresses: weeks 1 to 2 (gentle range of motion, symmetry work), weeks 3 to 6 (structured motion, manual therapy, lateral and protrusive exercises), and week 6+ (progressive diet advancement, functional retraining). Follow-up tracks MIO, excursions, pain, occlusal stability, and mechanical restriction. Plateau or recurrence warrants reassessment; suspected adhesions may benefit from arthroscopic lysis before escalating to open revision.

Clinical results

Table 5 summarizes published outcomes for the principal procedures described in this article.

Summary

Open TMJ surgery remains essential when structural pathology exceeds the limits of minimally invasive correction. Arthroscopic discopexy is the preferred approach for appropriately selected patients (Wilkes II–III, preserved disc morphology); open procedures—discopexy with Mitek anchor fixation, discectomy with interposition, arthroplasty, and eminectomy—are indispensable for advanced degeneration, disc nonviability, failed arthroscopy, or when concurrent osseous modification is required. Durable outcomes depend on disciplined preoperative selection, intraoperative disc assessment, conservative tissue handling, preservation of condylar height, and strict adherence to anatomic fascial planes during dissection. Early mobilization beginning within 24 to 48 hours and structured rehabilitation are essential determinants of long-term success and must be treated as integral components of the surgical plan.

Clinics care points

- Open temporomandibular joint surgery remains indispensable for advanced internal derangement and degenerative joint disease when structural pathology exceeds the limits of minimally invasive intervention.
- Disc preservation should be pursued only when morphology and mobility permit restoration of physiologic function; attempting to salvage nonviable discs increases morbidity and revision risk.
- Arthroscopic discopexy (McCain technique) is preferred for disc repositioning in Wilkes II to IV patients with preserved disc morphology and manageable adhesions; open discopexy is reserved for advanced disease, failed arthroscopy, or cases requiring concurrent open procedures.
- Open discopexy with Mitek Mini Anchor fixation: anchor placed 8 to 10 mm below the articular surface at the posterior-superior condylar head; 2 2-0 Ethibond sutures in horizontal mattress configuration through the posterior disc band.
- Preservation of condylar height, conservative arthroplasty, and subfascial dissection over the zygomatic arch are critical technical principles governing outcomes and neurologic safety.
- Early postoperative mobilization within 24 to 48 hours and structured rehabilitation are essential determinants of long-term success.

Declaration of AI and AI-assisted technologies in the writing process

During the preparation of this work, the authors used generative artificial intelligence tools (OpenAI ChatGPT and image-generation assistance) to create illustrations intended solely for educational visualization. All images were reviewed, edited, and verified by the authors. No AI-generated content was used to generate original research data, patient information, or diagnostic imaging. The authors take full responsibility for the accuracy, originality, and integrity of all text and figures included in this work.

Disclosure

The authors have nothing to disclose related to this article.

References

1. Renapurkar SK. Temporomandibular joint disc repositioning by suturing through open incision: a technical note. J Oral Maxillofac Surg 2018;76(5):948–54.
2. Al-Moraissi EA, Ellis E 3rd. Open versus arthroscopic surgery for the management of internal derangement of the temporomandibular joint: a meta-analysis. Int J Oral Maxillofac Surg 2015;44(7):763–70.
3. Sidebottom AJ. Current thinking in open temporomandibular joint surgery. Br J Oral Maxillofac Surg 2024;62.
4. Mehra P, Wolford LM. The mitek mini-anchor for TMJ disc repositioning: surgical technique and results. Int J Oral Maxillofac Surg 2001;30(6):497–503.
5. Marlière DAA, Vincentin Calori MJA, Medeiros YL, et al. Clinical outcomes of disc repositioning using suture anchors in TMJ internal derangement: a prospective evaluation. J Craniofac Surg 2023;34(1):e1–7.
6. Dolwick MF, Nitzan DW. TMJ disk surgery: 8-year Follow-Up evaluation. Fortschr Kiefer Gesichtschir 1990;35:162–3.
7. Montgomery MT, Gordon SM, Van Sickels JE, et al. Changes in signs and symptoms following temporomandibular joint disc repositioning surgery. J Oral Maxillofac Surg 1992;50(4):320–8.
8. Abramowicz S, Dolwick MF. Twenty-year Follow-Up study of disc repositioning surgery for TMJ internal derangement. J Oral Maxillofac Surg 2010;68(1):239–42.
9. Puthukkudiyil JS, Bhutia O, Roychoudhury A, et al. Does repositioning of the TMJ disc with bone anchors provide better outcomes than conventional plication? J Oral Maxillofac Surg 2020;78(11):2160–8.
10. McCain JP, Hossameldin RH, Srouji S, et al. Arthroscopic discopexy is effective in managing temporomandibular joint internal derangement in patients with wilkes stage II and III. J Oral Maxillofac Surg 2015;73(3):391–401.
11. McCain JP, Podrasky AE, Zabiegalski NA. Arthroscopic disc repositioning and suturing: a preliminary report. J Oral Maxillofac Surg 1992;50(4):568–79.
12. Holmlund AB, Gynther G, Axelsson S. Diskectomy in treatment of internal derangement of the temporomandibular joint: follow-up at 1, 3, and 5 years. Oral Surg Oral Med Oral Pathol 1993;76(2):266–71.
13. Eriksson L, Westesson PL. Long-term evaluation of meniscectomy of the temporomandibular joint. J Oral Maxillofac Surg 1985;43(4):263–9.

14. Takaku S, Toyoda T. Long-term evaluation of discectomy of the temporomandibular joint. J Oral Maxillofac Surg 1994;52(8): 722–6.
15.. Spallaccia F, De Tomaso S, Cirignaco G, et al. Temporo-mandibular joint functional arthroplasty: outcomes and indications. J Oral Maxillofac Surg 2025.
16.. Werkman DF, Mercuri L, Troost J, et al. An international survey on TMJ surgeons' implementation practices. J Craniomaxillofac Surg 2021;49.
17.. Warburton G, Patel N, Anchlia S, et al. Current treatment strategies for management of temporomandibular joint internal derangement with emphasis on arthroscopic surgery. J Clin Med 2021;10.
18. Badri O, Davis CM, Warburton G. Arthroscopic management and recent advancements in treatment of TMJ disorders. Br J Oral Maxillofac Surg 2024;62(9):820–5.
19. Israel HA. Technique for placement of a discal traction suture during temporomandibular joint arthroscopy. J Oral Maxillofac Surg 1989;47(3):311–3.
20. Kerstens HCJ, Tuinzing DB, van der Kwast WAM. Eminectomy and discoplasty for correction of the displaced temporomandibular joint disc. J Oral Maxillofac Surg 1989;47(2):150–4.

Autogenous and Alloplastic Reconstruction of the Temporomandibular Joint

Meshal Al Munif, DDS, SBOMFS [a,b], Clayton M. Davis, DDS, MD, MSc, FRCD(C) [c,*], Gary Warburton, DDS, MD, FDSRCS [d]

KEYWORDS

• Temporomandibular joint (TMJ) reconstruction • Alloplastic total joint replacement (TJR) • Autogenous grafts (costochondral graft) • Ankylosis and degenerative joint disease • Virtual surgical planning (VSP)

KEY POINTS

- Temporomandibular joint (TMJ) reconstruction restores mandibular function, occlusion, facial form, and airway support in conditions like ankylosis, trauma, and arthritis.
- Alloplastic total joint replacement is preferred in skeletally mature patients due to predictable outcomes and absence of donor-site morbidity.
- Autogenous grafts, particularly costochondral grafts, are favored in children due to growth potential but have variable outcomes.
- Custom TMJ prostheses allow precise anatomic restoration and are beneficial in complex deformities and revision cases.
- Virtual surgical planning enhances surgical accuracy, optimizing implant design, occlusion, and intraoperative execution.

Overview

Temporomandibular joint (TMJ) reconstruction is indicated in patients with joint destruction secondary to ankylosis, inflammatory or degenerative arthropathies, trauma, neoplasia, congenital deformity, or progressive condylar resorption. The goals of reconstruction are restoration of mandibular form and function, improvement in mastication, speech, airway support, and correction of occlusal and facial deformities. Surgical options include autogenous biologic reconstruction and alloplastic total joint replacement (TJR), each with subtypes and specific use cases. Technique selection is guided by patient age, pathology, prior surgery, and biomechanical considerations.[1,2]

General indications and contraindications

Indications

- *Bony or fibrous ankylosis* (especially recurrent ankylosis or large heterotopic bone masses) leading to near-complete jaw immobility.
- *End-stage degenerative joint disease*, such as advanced osteoarthritis or rheumatoid arthritis unresponsive to other treatments.
- *Failed previous joint reconstructions*, including failed autogenous grafts (eg, costochondral graft [CCG] resorption or ankylosis) or failed alloplastic implants.
- *Change in condylar–ramal height due to trauma, resorption, or neoplasia.*
- *Congenital or developmental abnormalities*, such as in hemifacial microsomia or idiopathic condylar resorption.[3]

In general, *alloplastic* TJR is favored in *skeletally mature* patients, it provides immediate restoration of joint function, avoids donor site morbidity, and yields more predictable long-term outcomes.[4] Modern TMJ alloplastic devices can be used to manage advanced disease with a reasonable expectation of achieving ~32 to 50 mm of postoperative opening and significant pain reduction.[5] In contrast, *autogenous reconstruction* is often preferred in *children or adolescents*, given the growth potential of autografts (especially CCGs) that can adapt with mandibular development.[4,6]

Contraindications

- *Active infection at the surgical site* is a strict contraindication—an infected field greatly increases the risk of implant failure and postoperative complications.
- *Allergy to implant materials*—True nickel or cobalt-chrome allergy, alternative using an all titanium prosthesis.[7]

[a] Faculty of Medicine and Dentistry, University of Alberta, Canada
[b] King Faisal Special Hospital and Research Centre, Riyadh, Saudi Arabia
[c] Faculty of Medicine and Dentistry, University of Alberta, Canada
[d] Department of Oral & Maxillofacial Surgery, University of Maryland School of Dentistry, Baltimore, MD, USA
* Corresponding author. Kingsway Oral Maxillofacial Surgery, 14310 111 Avenue Suite 107e, Edmonton, Alberta, T5M 3Z7, Canada.
E-mail address: cmd1@ualberta.ca

Atlas Oral Maxillofacial Surg Clin N Am 34 (2026) 235-245

https://doi.org/10.1016/j.cxom.2026.05.006
oralmaxsurgeryatlas.theclinics.com

Abbreviations

CCG	costochondral graft
CoCrMo	cobalt–chromium–molybdenum
MMF	maxillomandibular fixation
NSAIDs	nonsteroidal anti-inflammatory medication
TJR	total joint replacement
TMJ	temporomandibular joint
UHMWPE	ultrahigh-molecular-weight polyethylene

- *Severe systemic conditions that preclude major surgery* (for example, unstable cardiac disease or bleeding disorders) would also contraindicate an elective TMJ reconstruction.
- *Skeletal immaturity* is generally a relative contraindication for alloplastic joints, using a fixed-size device in a growing jaw can lead to secondary deformities; thus, autogenous options are usually recommended for young patients.[8] As more experience and success with TMJ TJR devices are gained and reported, the indications may include patients who have not achieved complete skeletal maturity. In some adolescent patients who have had severe ankylosis and multiple procedures, there is no potential for continued growth in the site of the ankylosed or mutilated joint[8]; therefore, TMJ TJR may be beneficial in limited cases such as children or adolescents with severe deformities.[9]
- *Psychological readiness* Careful counseling is essential for those unwilling or unable to participate in rehabilitation or those with psychiatric issues that affect compliance before joint reconstruction.

Autogenous reconstruction

Costochondral grafts

The CCG has historically been the most widely used autogenous option for TMJ reconstruction. Its popularity stems from ease of harvest, anatomic similarity to the mandibular condyle, and presumed growth potential in pediatric patients.[10]

Advantages

- Potential for adaptive growth in children
- Autogenous tissue with no foreign-body reaction
- Ability to reconstruct ramal height and joint continuity

Limitations

- Unpredictable growth (overgrowth or resorption)
- Ankylosis
- Donor-site morbidity
- Increased risk of failure in multiply operated joints or inflammatory conditions

Clinical series demonstrate variable long-term outcomes, particularly in adults and in joints with compromised vascular beds, where graft resorption and ankylosis remain significant concerns.[10]

Other autogenous options

Alternative biologic reconstructions include

- Sternoclavicular grafts
- Metatarsal graft
- Vascularized fibula flaps
- Iliac crest grafts
- Temporalis muscle or fascia flaps (primarily for interposition reconstruction)

Vascularized bone flaps provide improved graft survival in compromised beds but increase operative complexity and morbidity. Soft-tissue interposition alone does not reliably restore joint biomechanics in end-stage disease and is contraindicated in inflammatory arthropathies and multiply operated joints.[10,11]

Alloplastic total joint replacement

Alloplastic TJR provides immediate stability, eliminates donor-site morbidity, and offers predictable long-term outcomes. There are 2 types of alloplastic devices: custom (patient-specific) and stock (off-the-shelf).

Materials

TMJ total joint prostheses use cobalt–chromium–molybdenum (CoCrMo) alloys or titanium alloys for the condyle/ramus component and ultrahigh-molecular-weight polyethylene (UHMWPE) for the fossa. CoCrMo offers strong wear resistance but may trigger nickel hypersensitivity. Titanium alloys (Ti-6Al-4V) are biocompatible and corrosion-resistant, though rare hypersensitivity to aluminum and vanadium hypersensitivity can occur.

Manufacturing of alloplastic temporomandibular joint

Manufacturing relies on either subtractive milling or additive manufacturing (3D printing). Subtractive milling produces components with a refined, homogeneous grain structure and predictable mechanical strength. In contrast, 3D-printed titanium alloys often demonstrate needle-like, nonequilibrium microstructures, increased porosity, and less predictable corrosion and fatigue behavior. Current evidence supports milled components as the more dependable option for load-bearing TMJ prostheses.[12]

Custom alloplastic total joint replacement

Custom TMJ prostheses are designed using patient-specific computed tomography (CT) data and stereolithographic models. They allow precise restoration of mandibular position, ramal height, and occlusion, and are particularly advantageous in complex reconstructions.

Advantages

- Optimal fit and fixation
- Ability to address severe anatomic deformity

- Compatibility with simultaneous mandibular advancement orthognathic surgery

Stages of custom temporomandibular joint replacement

One-stage alloplastic TMJ total joint replacement involves resecting the diseased condyle and immediately placing of the alloplastic device in a single operation.

Indications
- Stable or correctable occlusion,
- Limited ankylosis,
- Preserved/minimally distorted fossa anatomy,
- Minimal need for skeletal or occlusal correction.

Two-stage alloplastic TMJ total joint replacement involves 2 procedures: the initial procedure to remove ankylosis or diseased bone, restore mandibular mobility, prepare the fossa, and place a temporary spacer, followed by the delayed second procedure to insert the definitive custom alloplastic device.

Indications
- Extensive bony ankylosis,
- Severe joint deformity,
- Large TMJ-region tumors,
- Failed prior reconstructions,
- Multiply operated joints requiring accurate postresection planning.

Preoperative planning

Virtual surgical planning

Step 1. Computed tomography acquisition (surgeon)
- Obtain a manufacturer-specific, medical-grade CT scan
  - Slice thickness: 0.5 to 1.0 mm
  - Zero gantry tilt
  - Coverage from at least 2.5 cm above the glenoid fossa to the inferior mandibular border
  - Maintain the correct occlusion during the CT scan

Step 2. Data submission to manufacturer (surgeon)
- Digital imaging and communications in medicine (DICOM) CT dataset obtained in the correct occlusion
- Dental anatomy data:
  - Intraoral scan (STL), laser-scanned stone models, or cone beam computed tomography (CBCT)-derived dental data

Step 3. Data processing and hybrid model generation (manufacturer/design engineer)
- Import CT DICOM data into proprietary planning software.
- Register dental anatomy to the skeletal dataset to eliminate artifact distortion.
- Generate a 1-piece hybrid craniofacial–dental 3-dimensional model with the mandible in the correct occlusion.
- Verify accuracy of occlusal and skeletal alignment before proceeding.

Step 4. Occlusal verification and mandibular positioning (Surgeon–Engineer collaboration)
- Confirm the final occlusion as scanned.
- Verify mandibular position relative to the cranial base.
- Confirm vertical ramus height and symmetry.
- Lock occlusion and mandibular position before bone resection planning.

Step 5. Virtual bone resection planning (design engineer with surgeon approval)
- Define the condylectomy level below the diseased condyle.
- Plan resection to achieve a joint gap typically measuring 15 to 20 mm.
- Identify the need for ipsilateral coronoidectomy.
- Plan removal of ankylotic or pathologic bone when present.
- Evaluate proximity to the cranial base, external auditory canal, and major vascular structures.
- Submit resection plan for surgeon review and approval.

Step 6. Custom alloplastic temporomandibular joint design (design engineer)
- Design patient-specific components using computer-aided design:
  - Fossa component: contoured to the temporal bone with appropriate bearing orientation
  - Mandibular component: restores ramus height and adapts to the lateral ramus
- Define:
  - Screw number, length, and orientation
  - Flange extension and component thickness

Step 7. Virtual plan review and final approval (surgeon)
- Review the complete virtual surgical plan, including:
  - Occlusion and mandibular position
  - Resection margins
  - Device design and articulation
  - Surgical guides cutting guides and guides with predictive holes Fig. 1

Step 8. Alloplastic temporomandibular joint fabrication (manufacturer)
- Manufacture custom mandibular and fossa components according to the approved plan.
- Perform quality control to confirm dimensional accuracy and surface integrity.
- Sterilize and package alloplastic device and guides for operative use.

Surgical technique

Step 1: patient positioning and presurgical preparation

- *Prophylactic intravenous antibiotics* are administered preoperatively.
- The patient is positioned *supine* and *nasally intubated.*
- *Short-acting neuromuscular blocking agents* are used during intubation to permit intraoperative facial nerve stimulation and identification.
- *Adequate ocular protection* is applied.
- The *external auditory canals* are irrigated with a *vancomycin solution* (1 g vancomycin in 1000 mL normal saline).
- Hair within the surgical field is shaved to approximately *1 cm above the ear helix* to ensure complete clearance from the operative field.
- A *head wrap* is applied to secure the endotracheal tube and isolate the patient's hair.
- The *face and neck* are prepared in the standard sterile fashion, with meticulous attention to minimizing contamination and maintaining sterility.
- After sterile draping, an *iodophor-impregnated sterile adhesive drape (Ioban, 3M)* is applied to cover the entire

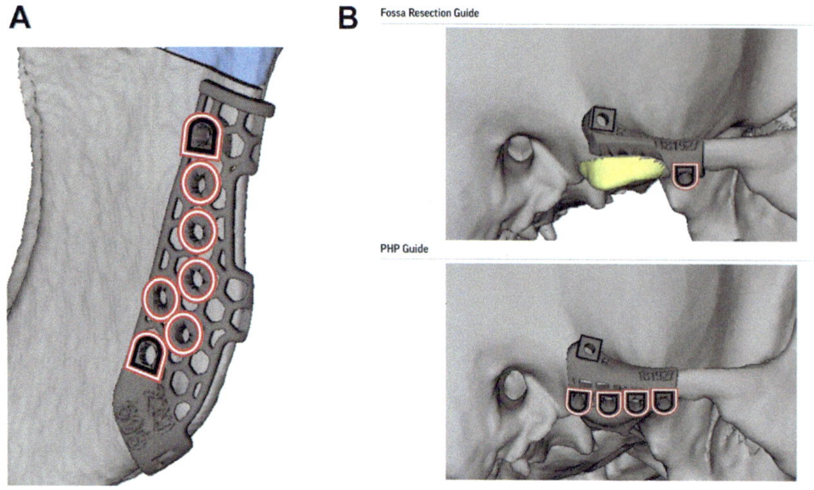

Fig. 1 (*A, B*) Surgical guides for ramus and fossa.

face and neck, isolating the mouth, nose, and endotracheal tube from the sterile field and creating a *watertight seal* to minimize salivary contamination during head rotation (Fig. 2).

- The head is then *tilted to the contralateral side*, and the adhesive drape is sharply incised with *Mayo scissors* to expose the ear, preauricular region, and retromandibular area.

Step 2: incision planning and surgical access

Surgical access is obtained through 2 incisions: a *modified retromandibular incision* for exposure of the mandibular ramus and an *endaural incision/invicision* for access to the TMJ (see Fig. 2).

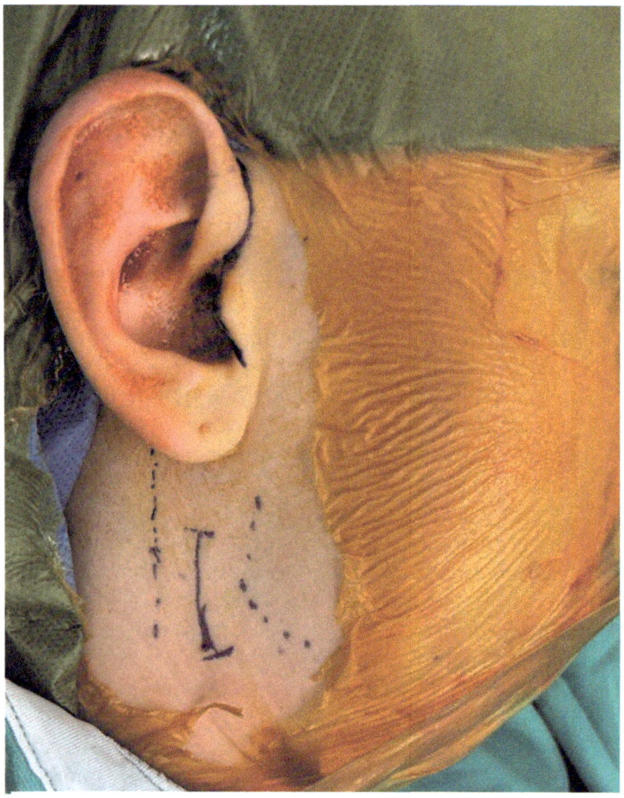

Fig. 2 Isolation of surgical field with Ioban dressing, endaural, and modified retromandibular incision markings.

1. Modified retromandibular incision

   Mark the anterior border of the sternocleidomastoid muscle, posterior border of the ramus, mandibular angle, and inferior border of the mandible. The incision is marked as a 3 to 4 cm curvilinear line, beginning approximately 1 fingerbreadth below the ear lobule and centered between the mandibular angle and the anterior border of the sternocleidomastoid muscle.

   The incision is carried through the skin and subcutaneous tissue to the platysma. The platysma is divided carefully, with a nerve stimulator used to identify and protect the marginal mandibular branch of the facial nerve. The plane between the parotid gland and masseter muscle is then developed.

   The superficial layer of the deep cervical fascia is opened vertically along the parotid-masseteric cleft. The parotid gland is retracted posteriorly, protecting the retromandibular vein and facial nerve branches. A nerve stimulator may be used throughout the dissection to confirm the location of facial nerve branches.

   The pterygomasseteric sling and periosteum are incised along the mandibular angle and inferior border. Subperiosteal dissection is then performed to expose the lateral and posterior ramus, inferior border, sigmoid notch, and condylar neck (Fig. 3).

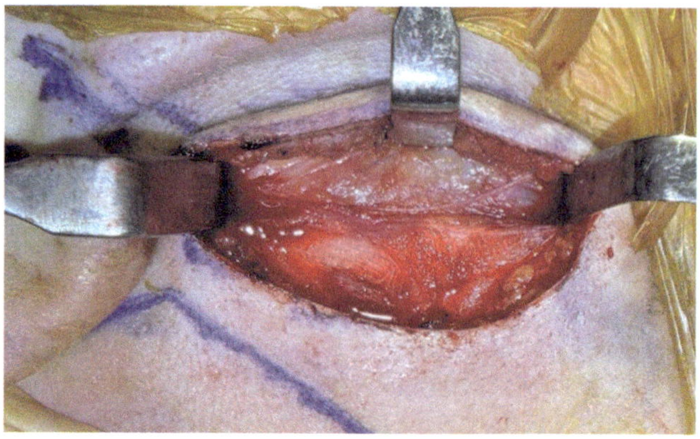

Fig. 3 Marginal mandibular branches of facial nerve.

2. The endaural incision/invcision
   Mark the incision from the superior auricular crease between the helix and preauricular skin, extending inferiorly toward the intertragal notch, with the central portion hidden behind the tragal edge.
   Carry the incision through the skin and subcutaneous tissue. Dissection is developed in relation to the zygomatic arch. Inferior to the arch, perform blunt dissection in the avascular plane anterior to the tragal cartilage and external auditory canal to create a pocket. Superior to the arch, continue dissection until the smooth, white superficial temporalis fascia is identified. Place a self-retaining retractor for exposure.
   Incise the superficial layer of the deep temporal fascia vertically for approximately 2 cm down to the zygomatic arch. Continue subperiosteal dissection anteriorly along the arch using a periosteal elevator. The superficial temporal vessels, if encountered, are ligated or gently retracted anteriorly.
   This plane protects the facial nerve branches and permits anterior retraction of the soft tissues. Release the posterior attachment of the parotideomasseteric fascia just anterior to the external auditory canal to expose the lateral TMJ capsule.
   Open the superior capsule to enter the glenoid fossa. Use a Freer elevator to separate the capsule from the lateral condyle and then make a vertical capsular incision to expose the condylar neck and condyloid process.
   Now, the 2 surgical planes are connected, providing full exposure of the joint capsule, zygomatic arch, articular eminence, condylar neck, and the entire lateral surface of the mandibular ramus.

Step 3: condylectomy

1. Retractor placement
   Place 2 Dunn-Dautrey retractors: one anteriorly in the sigmoid notch and one posteriorly behind the condylar neck. Both retractors should engage the medial surface of the condyle to protect the internal maxillary artery, masseteric vessels, and inferior alveolar nerve (Fig. 4).
2. First osteotomy: condylar head removal
   Perform the initial condylectomy at the condylar neck without the guide. A piezosurgery device is used to minimize the risk of vascular injury. Remove the condylar head to allow superior mobilization of the remaining condylar neck and ramus, improving visualization (Fig. 5).

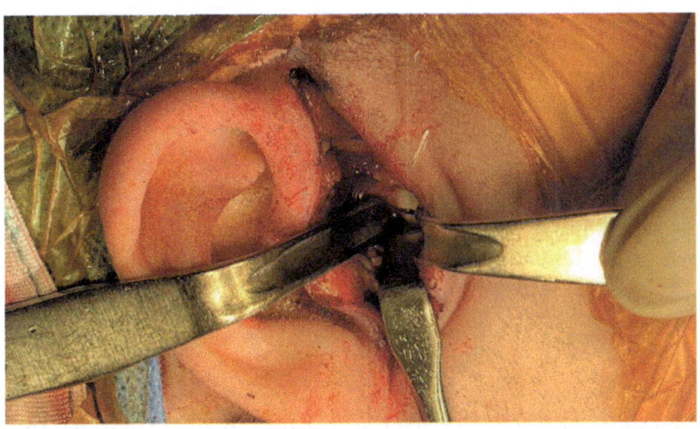

Fig. 4 Condylar Retractors (Dunn-Dautrey) and condylectomy.

3. Second osteotomy: definitive guided cut
   Seat the virtual surgical planning (VSP)-derived ramal cutting guide on the lateral surface of the mandibular ramus and secure it with 2 screws. Perform the definitive second osteotomy at the planned level. This prevents residual bony interference and ensures optimal adaptation and contact of the ramal component (Fig. 6).
   Predictive-hole guides may be used to guide implant positioning and reduce or eliminate the need for maxillomandibular fixation (MMF).
4. Clearance check
   After removal of the remaining condylar segment, confirm adequate clearance between the ramal osteotomy and the articular eminence/fossa region to accommodate both the fossa and ramal components without interference.
5. Guide removal
   Remove the ramal cutting guide

Step 4: glenoid fossa preparation

1. *Complete discectomy:* The articular disc and posterior attachment tissue are excised completely and sent for pathologic.
2. *Debridement:* All synovial tissue, granulation tissue, fibrous adhesions, and heterotopic bone are removed using curettes, rongeurs, and a piezosurgery device. In ankylosis cases, the ankylotic bony mass is removed from the fossa floor and surrounding structures until the native fossa contour is identified. A VSP-derived fossa cutting guide may be used when available (see Fig. 1).
3. *Articular eminence management:* The articular eminence is assessed relative to the planned fossa component position. Any prominence that prevents flush seating is reduced with a piezosurgery device or osteotome under direct vision.
4. *Hemostasis and irrigation:* Hemostasis is achieved with bone wax, electrocautery, and topical hemostatic agents such as thrombin, collagen, or oxidized cellulose. The fossa is then thoroughly irrigated before implant trialing or placement.

Step 5: coronoidectomy

- Coronoidectomy, if required, is performed through the endaural approach at this stage.
- Indications for coronoidectomy include:
  1. Impingement of the coronoid process on the posterior zygomatic body following significant mandibular advancement,
  2. Persistent limitation in mouth opening due to temporalis muscle-tendon shortening, as commonly encountered in ankylosis cases, despite completion of the condylectomy.

Step 6: *setting the occlusion ± intermediate splint* (this step is avoided if predictive hole guides are used)

- *Transition from the sterile temporomandibular joint replacement (TMJR) field to the contaminated oral cavity* is required to establish the planned occlusion using the *VSP-derived intermediate splint*.
- A *separate Mayo stand* with dedicated intraoral and *MMF instruments* is prepared to prevent contamination of the sterile instruments used for insertion and fixation of the TMJR components.

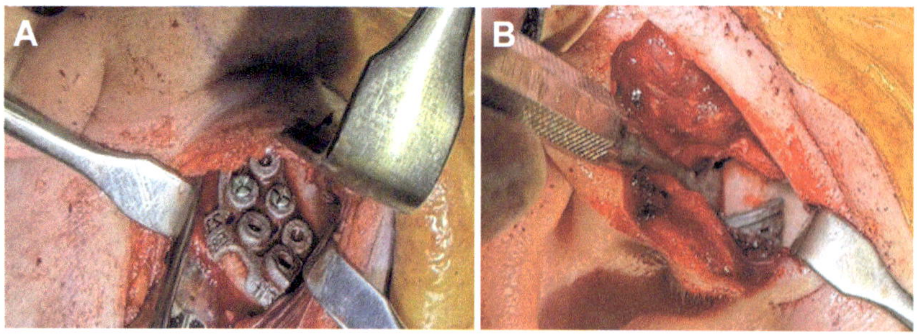

Fig. 5 (*A*, *B*) Condylar osteotomy guide for TJR placed on mandible (*right side*).

- Before entering the oral cavity, the *sterile field is isolated* using a *new split-sheet drape* covering the entire patient and leaving only the oral cavity exposed.
- The *loban adhesive drape* is incised to allow access to the oral cavity.
- In cases involving a *unilateral alloplastic joint with a contralateral sagittal split osteotomy*, the sagittal split is performed at this stage using instruments set up on the intraoral Mayo stand.
- The occlusion is established using an *intermediate splint* if the occlusion is not stable, and the patient is secured into the planned occlusion using *orthodontic hooks or MMF screws.*
- After verification of a stable occlusion, strict measures are taken to *re-establish sterility.*
- The *split-sheet drape and towels* are removed, and the surgeon and assistants *change gowns and gloves.*
- A *new loban adhesive drape* is applied to completely isolate the oral cavity and cover all previously exposed and contaminated areas, ensuring a clean sterile field before continuation of the TMJR procedure.

Step 7: *implantation of the alloplastic devices*

- The *surgical sites are irrigated thoroughly* with copious amounts of the prepared *vancomycin solution and sterile betadine* before seating of the TMJR components.
- The *TMJR fossa component* is seated in its planned position and *fixated first*, followed by seating of the *ramal component.*
- Care is taken throughout component placement to *minimize contact with the skin* during insertion of the components.
- Proper seating of the *TMJR condylar head* is confirmed when it is centered mediolaterally within the fossa component bearing surface and positioned firmly against the *posterior stop* of the fossa component (Figs. 7 and 8).
- Any deviation from the planned position, as defined by the *VSP schematics and stereolithographic model*, suggests *bony and/or soft tissue interference* and must be identified and corrected before fixation.
- Once correct positioning is confirmed, the *ramal component is fixated* using the *preplanned bicortical screw length* specified on the planning schematics.

Finite element analysis has demonstrated that the most superior ramal component fixation screw carries the greatest load. Therefore, even though it can sometimes be difficult to access this hole for screw placement, it is an important screw biomechanically.[13]

Use the screw lengths provided on the planning schematic. TMJR ramal component fixation screws that are too long can

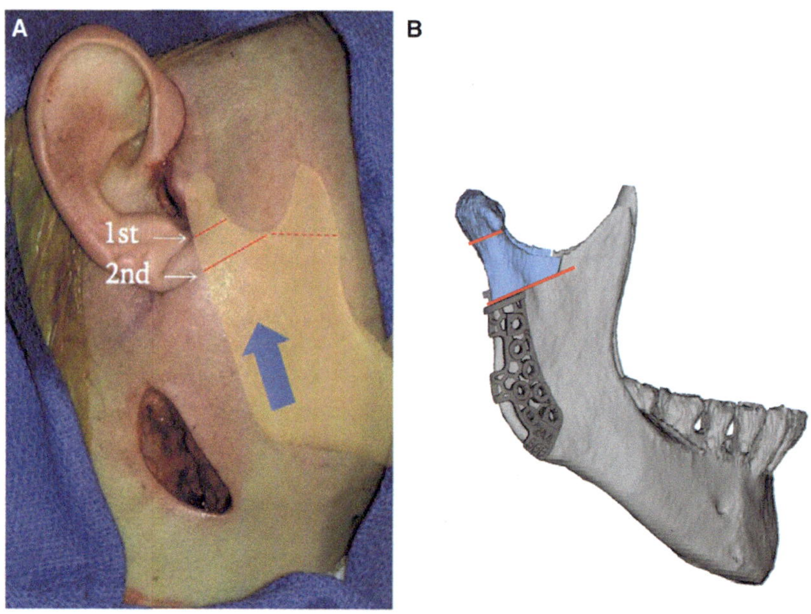

Fig. 6 (*A*, *B*) First and second condylar osteotomy mark. Push the mandible superiorly to gain better access for the 2nd osteotomy (*blue arrow*).

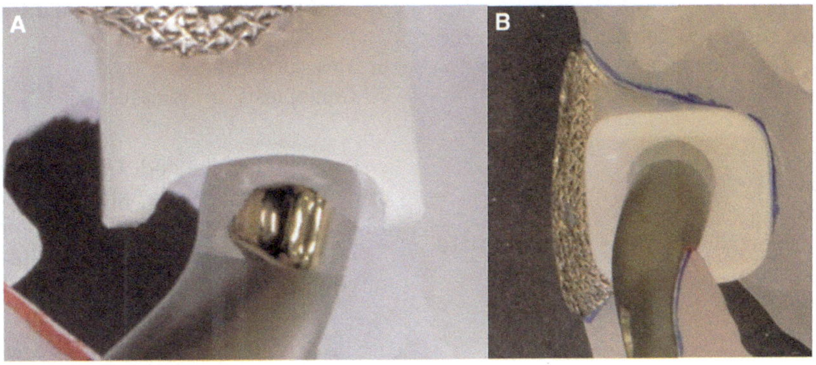

Fig. 7 (*A, B*) Correct positioning of condylar component superior posterior position in middle of fossa.

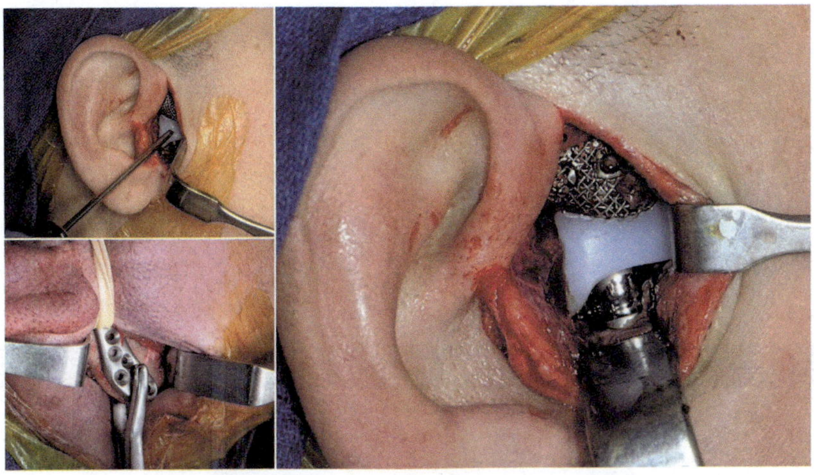

Fig. 8 Correct positioning of condylar component.

penetrate the medial pterygoid muscle and be a source of muscle injury, fibrosis, and pain during function.[14]

Step 8: closure of the surgical sites

The incisions are irrigated *vancomycin solution and sterile betadine. Vancomycin powder can be applied just before* closure (Fig. 9).

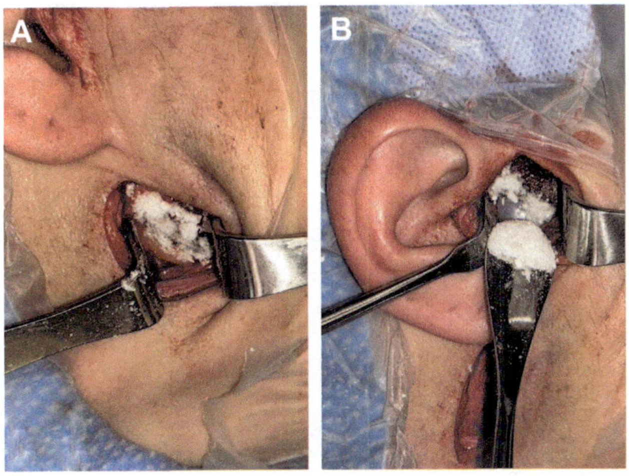

Fig. 9 (*A, B*) Vancomycin powder over fossa and condyle.

Closure of retromandibular wound: The parotid fascia and capsule are closed with 3-0 resorbable sutures to reduce the risk of sialocele and salivary fistula formation. The subcutaneous tissue is closed with 3-0 resorbable sutures to eliminate dead space. Skin is closed with 5-0 monofilament sutures.

Closure of endaural wound: The temporal fascia and superficial temporal fascia are reapproximated to the anterior capsule remnants or periosteum with 3-0 resorbable sutures. The subcutaneous and subcartilaginous layers of the endaural incision are closed with 3-0 resorbable sutures. Skin is closed with 5-0 monofilament sutures.

A pressure dressing is applied and kept on for 24 hours. Full range of motion testing is performed at the end of the case to check for any dislocation tendency. Guiding elastics may be placed for immediate postoperative comfort and to prevent condylar sag or dislocation.

Combine custom TMJR with other reconstructive surgeries

Combine TMJR and orthognathic

This procedure is used when the TMJR is needed and the patient also has dentofacial deformities that requiring orthognathic surgery.

Virtual surgical planning

The VSP for the orthognathic surgery is completed first in the standard planning fashion. The recommended sequence for orthognathic VSP is

1. Maxillary midline correction
2. Maxillary cant correction
3. Advancement of the maxilla
4. Vertical correction of the maxilla to provide appropriate incisor show with lips in repose
5. Occlusal plane correction via differential impaction or down graft
6. Yaw correction
7. Genioplasty if indicated

Finally, the planned TMJR condylectomies are completed using the VSP software, allowing a sufficient vertical space of 13 to 15 mm for the alloplastic components.[14]

After completing the VSP, occlusal splints for orthognathic surgery and a stereolithographic model for TMJR fabrication

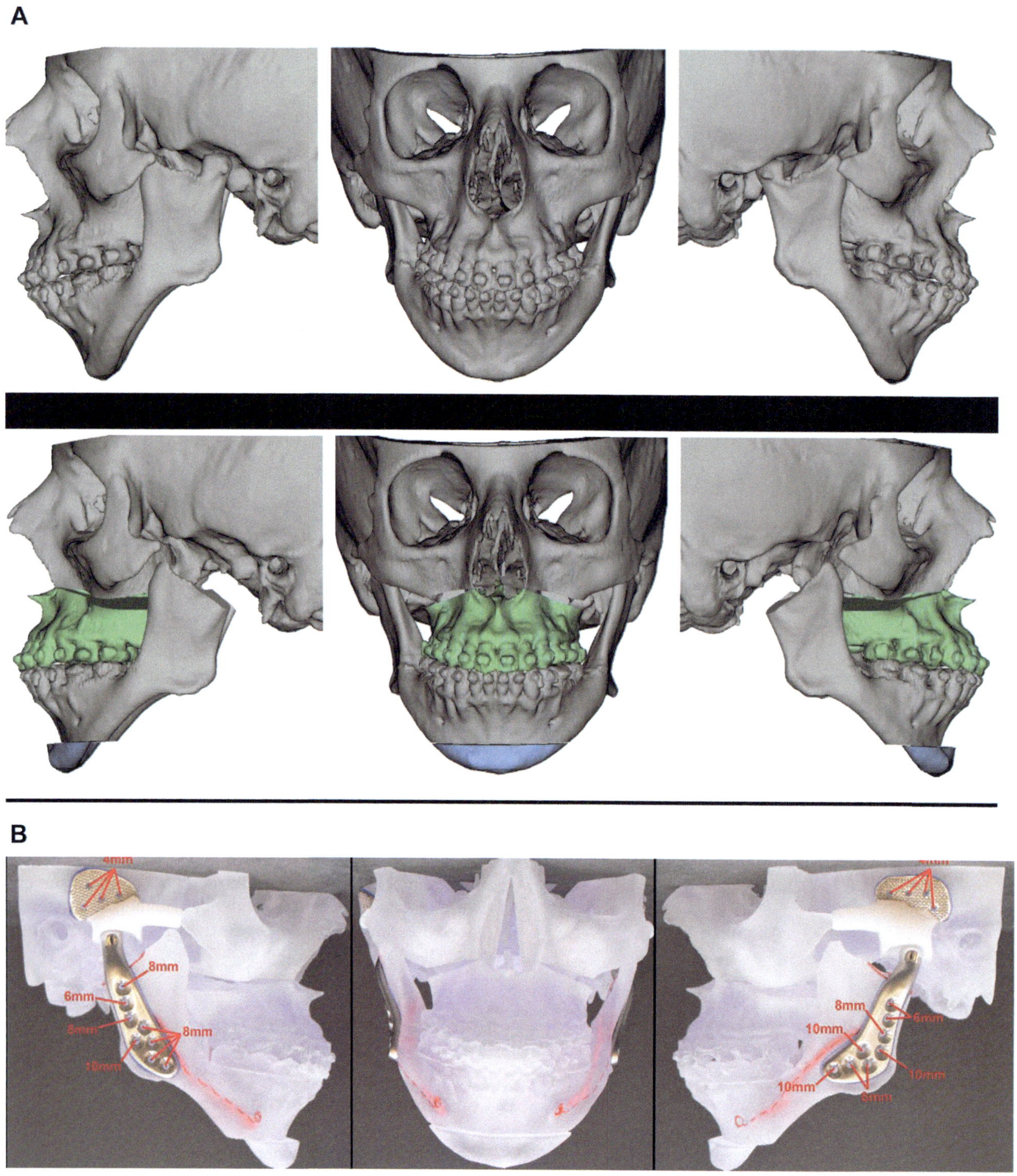

Fig. 10 (*A, B*) VSP surgical planning for Lefort Bilateral extended temporomandibular joint replacement (eTJR) and genioplasty.

are created from the same data. This data can also be sent digitally to the device manufacturer for designing and manufacturing a custom TMJR device. The device design can then be used to fabricate cutting guides with predictive holes.

When planning a significant advancement using a TMJR device, check if the coronoid will impinge on the zygoma using VSP. If impingement is seen, include coronoidectomies in the surgical plan (Fig. 10).

Sequencing of the surgical procedure

It is recommended to perform the TMJR portion of the surgery first and then complete the orthognathic procedures second. This approach is recommended for 2 reasons:

1. Minimizes the risk of contamination of the sterile TMJR surgical site from the oral cavity.
2. When there has been vertical shortening of the posterior ramus and condyle (eg, condylar resorption, trauma malunions, or congenital conditions) and the maxillary occlusal plane is steep as a result, space must first be created by restoring the vertical height with the TMJR to move the posterior maxilla down.

Stock temporomandibular joint replacement

The Stock prostheses are prefabricated systems (off-the-shelf) designed to fit a range of anatomic variations. They are cost-effective, readily available, and suitable for patients with relatively preserved anatomy.

Prothesis design and sizes

Stock TJR systems, like the Biomet TMJ Replacement System, use standardized sizes to fit various patient anatomies. The mandibular component is made from a cobalt-chrome alloy (ASTM type F799) plasma-sprayed with a roughened titanium coating on the medial host bone side of the ramal plate. It comes in 3 ramus lengths (45 mm, 50 mm, 55 mm) and multiple geometries (standard, narrow, offset) to accommodate asymmetries. The UHMWPE fossa component is available in 3 sizes, with only the anterior-posterior length of the zygomatic flange varying, allowing for multiple screw fixation sites. The articulating surface of the fossa has the same geometric configuration and dimensions in 3 sizes, all with the same curvature to articulate with any condylar size[9] (Fig. 11).

Surgical preparation for stock total joint replacement

Similar surgical exposure and resection of the TMJ as early discussed in custom TMJ TJR, the differences are

- *Fossa placement*: Begin by selecting the appropriate fossa size. To ensure stable fossa placement, surgically flatten the articular eminence with a reciprocating diamond rasp whose cutting depth matches the alloplastic fossa component.
- *Condylar Component Placement:* With the patient in intermaxillary fixation, one of 3 condylar sizers (45, 50, or 55 mm) is used to confirm proper fit between the fossa and condylar prostheses. A diamond reciprocating rasp smooths lateral ramus irregularities to ensure a flush fit of the device. The condylar head should be positioned as posteriorly as possible to allow some pseudotranslation.

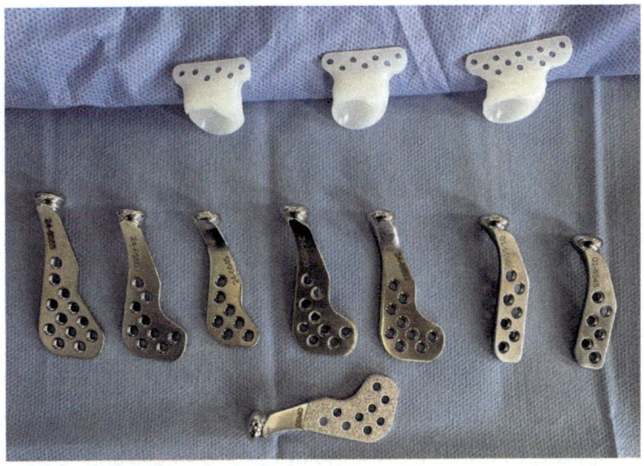

Fig. 11 Stock TJR components with varying sizes of fossa and condylar component.

- Many surgeons *provisionally fixate each component* with 2 screws in each before checking function. This allows for alteration of the position if necessary and still having good bone for fixation.

Virtual surgical planning can be used to plan surgery with a prefabricated stock TMJ device. It helps choose the appropriate prosthetic size and determine the amount of host bone modification needed. It also aids in fabricating surgical guides to place the stock TMJ TJR components.[15]

Complications and management

Intraoperative complications

- *Bleeding*: usually arises from the middle meningeal, internal maxillary, or masseteric arteries, or the lateral pterygoid muscles. Vessel ligation is preferred but challenging. Hemostatic agents like thrombin, collagen, or flow seal help control bleeding. For severe bleeding, the external carotid can be accessed via a retromandibular incision, and interventional radiology may be used to locate and occlude the vessel.
- *Facial nerve injury*: Careful dissection and judicious retraction minimize the risk of facial nerve injury. Nerve monitoring may be used for complex cases with distorted anatomy.

Early complications

- *Dislocation:* Immediate postoperative dislocation can be managed by manual reduction and placement of intermaxillary elastics for 3 weeks. Late dislocation may require sedation and/or general anesthetic in combination with manual reduction, or possible surgical intervention to achieve relocation. This is more frequent in patients with concomitant coronoidectomies.
- *Infection*: Prosthetic joint infection rates are ~2.5%. Prosthetic infection can be difficult to treat, often secondary to the formation of a biofilm. Early (acute) infections within 3 to 4 weeks can potentially be salvaged, and managed with wound washout, debridement, and irrigation, followed by 4 to 6 weeks of IV therapy. Chronic (late) infections require explantation and insertion of an antibiotic impregnated

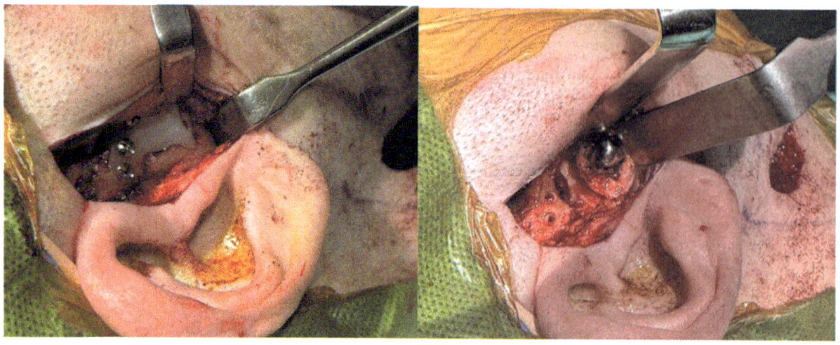

Fig. 12 Heterotopic bone surrounding TMJ prosthesis.

spacer, followed by IV antibiotics for 6 weeks and replacement of the device after 8 to 10 weeks.[16]

- *Hematoma*: Increases risk of infection and may require drainage.
- *Nerve Injury*: Facial nerve branches (temporal and marginal mandibular) are at risk during dissection and retraction but often recover spontaneously.
- *Malocclusion*: Improper condylar seating or fibrous tension can cause this condition. Minor discrepancies usually resolve on their own, but severe cases may require refixation or postoperative adjustment.
- *Pain*: May result from muscle spasm or inflammation and is typically managed with analgesics and early physiotherapy.

Late complications (months to years postop) include

- *Heterotopic bone formation and re-ankylosis*: Heterotopic bone formation is most common in patients with ankylotic conditions or those who have undergone multiple surgeries (Fig. 12).

Several methods can help prevent this complication:

- Autogenous fat grafting around the prosthetic joint.[17]
- Nonsteroidal anti-inflammatory medication (NSAIDs), such as indomethacin.[18]
- Low-dose postoperative irradiation, with reported regimens including 10 Gy given in 5 daily fractionated doses during the immediate postoperative period.[19,20]
- *Prosthetic Loosening or Wear*: Rare with modern designs; screw loosening may be monitored or revised if symptomatic.
- *Allergic Reactions*: Hypersensitivity to metals like nickel; preop screening and hypoallergenic options are preventive strategies.
- *Adjacent Structure Degeneration*: Occlusal changes and opposite joint wear may develop and require long-term monitoring.
- *Revision Surgery*: Indicated for persistent pain, infection, component failure, or reankylosis; occurs in ~3 to 5% of cases.

Rehabilitation and recovery

- Perioperative antibiotics are administered, typically a first-generation cephalosporin.
- Many surgeons continue oral antibiotics for 7 to 10 days postoperatively. However, the literature supports just 24 hours of perioperative antibiotics.
- Tight elastic MMF is maintained for 1 week, followed by light elastic MMF for an additional 2 weeks.
- Active and passive range-of-motion exercises are initiated at postoperative Week 3, coinciding with removal of the elastics.
- Rehabilitation includes stretching exercises performed four times daily to progressively increase maximum incisal opening.
- Patients are maintained on a soft, nonchew diet for 6 weeks postoperatively.

Clinics care points

- Patient selection is the most important determinant of successful temporomandibular joint reconstruction; treatment choice should be guided by age, pathology, prior surgery, skeletal maturity, and functional goals.

- Alloplastic total joint replacement is preferred patients because it provides predictable restoration of function, avoids donor-site morbidity, and produces reliable long-term outcomes.
- High-resolution CT imaging and meticulous virtual surgical planning are critical for accurate prosthesis design, restoration of ramal height, occlusion, and improve accuracy of prosthesis placement.
- Predictive-hole cutting guides may improve operative efficiency and reduce the need for intraoperative maxillomandibular fixation.
- Proper superior-posterior seating of the condylar component within the fossa is essential; malposition should prompt evaluation for residual bony or soft-tissue interference before fixation.
- The most superior fixation screw of the ramal component carries the highest biomechanical load and should be prioritized during fixation whenever possible.
- Heterotopic bone formation remains an important late complication, particularly in ankylosis and multiply operated joints; consideration should be given to preventive strategies including fat grafting, nonsteroidal anti-inflammatory medications, and selected postoperative radiation protocols.
- Early rehabilitation with structured range-of-motion exercises is critical to optimize postoperative function and improve maximal incisal opening.

References

1. Mercuri LG. Alloplastic temporomandibular joint replacement: rationale for the use of custom devices. Int J Oral Maxillofac Surg 2012;41:1033–40.
2. Lindqvist C, Jokinen J, Paukku P, et al. Adaptation of autogenous costochondral grafts used for temporomandibular joint reconstruction: a long-term clinical and radiologic follow-up. J Oral Maxillofac Surg 1988;46:465–70.
3. Henry CH, Wolford LM. Treatment outcomes for temporomandibular joint reconstruction after failed proplast-teflon implant failed. J Oral Maxillofac Surg 1993;51:352.
4. Leandro LFL, Ono HY, Loureiro CCDS, et al. A 10-year experience and follow-up of 300 patients with the Biomet/Lorenz Microfixation TMJ replacement system. Int J Oral Maxillofac Surg 2013;42:1007.
5. Voiner J, Yu J, Deitrich P, et al. Analysis of mandibular motion following unilateral and bilateral alloplastic TMJ reconstruction. Int J Oral Maxillofac Surg 2011;40:569–71.
6. MacIntosh RB. The case for autogenous reconstruction of the adult temporomandibular joint. In: Worthington P, Evans JR, editors. Controversies in oral and maxillofacial surgery. Philadelphia: WB Saunders; 1994. p. 356–80.
7. Mercuri LG, Alcheikh Ali F, Woolson R. Outcomes of total alloplastic replacement with peri-articular autogenous fat grafting for management of re-ankylosis of the temporomandibular joint. J Oral Maxillofac Surg 2008;66:1794.
8. Mercuri LG, Swift JQ. Considerations for the use of alloplastic temporomandibular joint replacement in the growing patient. J Oral Maxillofac Surg 2009;67:1979–90.
9. Quinn PD, Granquist EJ. Atlas of temporomandibular joint surgery. 2nd edition. Hoboken (NJ): Wiley-Blackwell; 2015. Chapter 5.
10. Kent JN, Haggerty CJ. Autogenous reconstruction of the temporomandibular joint. In: Atlas of operative oral and maxillofacial surgery.
11. Quinn PD. Alloplastic reconstruction of the temporomandibular joint: selected readings on oral and maxillofacial surgery. Selected Readings in Oral and Maxillofacial Surgery 1999;7(5):1–20.
12. Mercuri LG, Neto MQ, Pourzal R. Alloplastic temporomandibular joint replacement: present status and future perspectives of the elements of embodiment. Int J Oral Maxillofac Surg 2022;51(12):1573–8.
13. Arabshahi Z, Kadir MRA, Koloor SSR, et al. Finite element analysis of temporomandibular joint implant under fi ve simulated clenching loads. Adv Sci Lett 2013;19(11):3293–6.
14. Warburton G, Mercuri LG. Alloplastic reconstruction of the temporomandibular joint in patients with dentofacial deformities. Atlas Oral Maxillofac Surg Clin North Am 2022;30(2):223–33.
15. Chandran R, Keeler GD, Christensen AM, et al. Application of virtual surgical planning for total joint reconstruction with a stock alloplast system. J Oral Maxillofac Surg 2011;69:285–94.
16. Wolford LM, Rodrigues DB, McPhillips A. Management of the infected temporomandibular joint total joint prosthesis. J Oral Maxillofac Surg 2010;68:2810.
17. Wolford LM, Karras SC. Autologous fat transplantation around temporomandibular joint total joint prostheses: preliminary treatment outcomes. J Oral Maxillofac Surg 1997;55:245.
18. Kienapfel H, Koller M, Wust A, et al. Prevention of heterotopic bone formation after total hip arthroplasty. Arch Orthop Trauma Surg 1999;119:292.
19. Durr ED, Turlington EG, Foote RL. Radiation treatment of heterotopic bone formation in the temporomandibular articulation. Int J Radiat Oncol Biol Phys 1993;27:863.
20. Reid R, Cooke H. Postoperative ionizing radiation in the management of heterotopic bone formation in the temporomandibular joint. J Oral Maxillofac Surg 1999;57:900.

Pathology of the Temporomandibular Joint

Hyperplasia, Neoplasms, and Resection

Adit Gadh, DMD [a,*], Daniel Choi, DDS, MD [b], David Joey Chang, DMD [c]

KEYWORDS

- Temporomandibular joint • Condylar hyperplasia • Osteochondroma • Calcified chondroid mesenchymal neoplasm • Pigmented villonodular synovitis • Condylectomy • TMJ resection • Total joint replacement

KEY POINTS

- Management of temporomandibular joint (TMJ) pathology rests on 3 principles: confirm biologic behavior, completely remove the growth center or tumor, and restore mandibular form and function.
- High condylectomy is the primary treatment for active condylar hyperplasia and selected benign condylar lesions; proportional condylectomy with virtual surgical planning can achieve single-stage symmetry.
- Osteochondroma is the most common benign TMJ tumor; resection level is dictated by structural involvement of the condylar head, not tumor size.
- Synovial, crystalline, and proliferative TMJ lesions are benign but locally aggressive, may involve the skull base, are often diagnosed arthroscopically, and are definitively treated with total joint replacement.
- Malignant lesions require margin-negative en bloc resection; reconstruction is individualized and selected at the planning stage.

Introduction

Pathologic conditions of the temporomandibular joint (TMJ) that require surgical resection are uncommon but demand a management strategy distinct from internal derangement or degenerative joint disease. Most are structural and progressive: condylar hyperplasia (CH) and benign condylar tumors such as osteochondroma alter mandibular growth, occlusion, and facial symmetry, while malignant tumors, though rare, mandate oncologic resection with immediate reconstruction. The surgeon's task is not simply to relieve symptoms but to determine biologic activity, define resection margins, and restore mandibular height and occlusal stability. Management rests on 3 principles: accurate diagnosis and confirmation of biologic behavior; complete removal of the pathologic growth center or tumor; and restoration of mandibular form, function, and occlusion. This chapter is organized by pathology—hyperplasia, benign neoplasms, and malignancy—and pairs each entity with its treatment algorithm and operative pearls. Because the surgical corridor is largely shared across these conditions, access is considered first.

[a] Endoscopic Maxillofacial Surgery, Oral and Maxillofacial Surgery, Massachusetts General Hospital, Boston, MA, USA
[b] Oral and Maxillofacial Surgery, Massachusetts General Hospital, Boston, MA, USA
[c] Oral and Maxillofacial Surgery, Tufts University, Boston, MA, USA
* Corresponding author. Oral and Maxillofacial Surgery, Massachusetts General Hospital, 55 Fruit Street, Unit 230, Boston, MA 02114.
E-mail address: agadh@mgh.harvard.edu

Surgical access: open versus endoscopic approaches

Access to the TMJ can be obtained through either an extraoral or an intraoral corridor. The choice is determined by surgeon experience, anatomic considerations, and case complexity rather than by any difference in resection principles; the completeness and orientation of the resection take precedence over the incision.[1] Two approaches are described here: the standard preauricular approach, and the endoscopic-assisted intraoral approach—a contemporary alternative for selected condylectomies that we use at our institution.

Extraoral preauricular approach

1. Incision: Preauricular crease incision anterior to the tragus from the helical root to the tragal base; extend as an inverted hockey-stick into the temporal hairline for greater superior exposure. Endaural or *inviscision* variants may be used for esthetic preference.
2. Dissection planes: Develop 2 connected planes—superiorly, deep to the temporoparietal fascia down to the temporalis fascia; inferiorly, on the avascular, nerve-free tragal perichondrium directly to the lateral capsule. The tragal pointer confirms the facial nerve (~1 cm deep, ~1 cm inferior).
3. Zygomatic arch exposure: Incise temporalis fascia and muscle to bone and elevate subperiosteally over the lateral arch—the principal facial nerve protection maneuver—to

1061-3315/26/
https://doi.org/10.1016/j.cxom.2026.05.010
oralmaxsurgeryatlas.theclinics.com

Abbreviations

CCMN	calcified chondroid mesenchymal neoplasm
CH	condylar hyperplasia
PVMN	pigmented villonodular synovitis
TMJ	temporomandibular joint
VSP	virtual surgical planning

reach the articular eminence. Palpate the condyle before entering the joint to avoid the external auditory canal and middle ear.

4. Capsular entry. After elevating the parotid off the capsule, make a T-shaped capsulotomy; the horizontal limb over the eminence exposes the superior space and a lateral limb exposes the inferior space when disc access is required. Place a malleable retractor medial to the neck to protect the maxillary artery, pterygoid venous plexus, and middle cranial fossa.
5. Closure. Reapproximate capsule, periosteum, fascia, subcutis, and skin in layers; pressure dressing for 24 hours.

Endoscopic-assisted intraoral approach

This approach provides direct line-of-sight access to the condyle through an intraoral incision, eliminates the facial scar, and reduces risk to the facial nerve. It is best suited to high and proportional condylectomy for hyperplasia and to small, superiorly based osteochondromas, and is not appropriate for oncologic resection or for lesions requiring access to the fossa or skull base.

1. Incision: Vestibular incision along the external oblique ridge from mid-ramus to the first molar.
2. Exposure: Subperiosteal dissection of the lateral ramus, sigmoid notch, and coronoid base.
3. Coronoidectomy: Strip the temporalis from the coronoid and osteotomize it at its base, removing it to create a direct corridor to the condylar head.
4. Endoscopic orientation: Advance a rigid endoscope (2.7 mm, 0°, or 30°) along the medial ramus to visualize the medial and posterior surfaces inaccessible to direct view.
5. Guide placement: Seat the virtual surgical planning (VSP)–derived patient-specific cutting guide on the condylar head and confirm circumferential seating endoscopically, with particular attention to the medial pole; provisionally fixate (Figs. 1 and 2).
6. Osteotomy: Position a malleable retractor medial to the condylar neck, then cut through the guide slot under endoscopic visualization, preserving the medial cortex.
7. Specimen and hemostasis: Release the lateral pterygoid, deliver the specimen intraorally (in 2 pieces if large), and control bleeding with packing, bipolar cautery, and topical hemostatic agent; remain mindful of the masseteric, pterygoid, and internal maxillary vessels.
8. Closure: Resorbable closure of the vestibular incision; the coronoid is not replaced. If circumferential guide seating or the osteotomy cannot be completed safely, convert to the extraoral approach (Fig. 3).

Pearl: Approach selection should never compromise the completeness or orientation of the resection; visualization and precision take precedence over incision choice.[1]

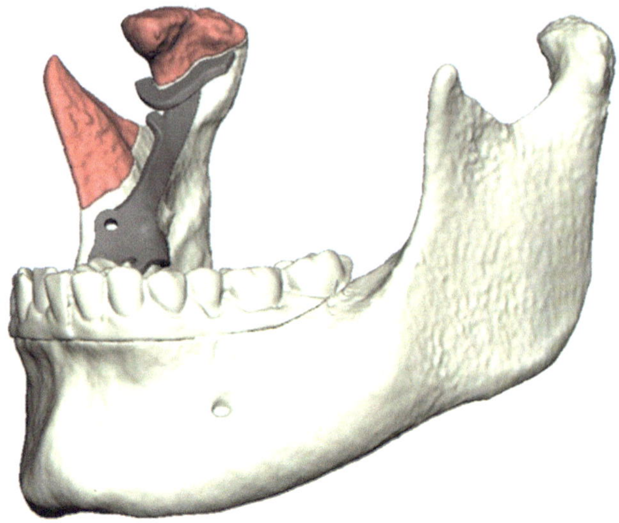

Fig. 1 Computer-aided design of surgical guide to direct the proportional condylectomy via intraoral approach.

Condylar hyperplasia

CH is a pathologic overgrowth of the mandibular condyle producing progressive facial asymmetry, occlusal canting, chin deviation, and functional imbalance.[2] Although it may resemble dentofacial deformity, the condyle behaves as an active growth center, and failure to address ongoing hyperactivity produces continued asymmetry even after orthodontic or orthognathic treatment.[3] The central management question is whether growth remains active.

Preoperative evaluation and planning

Activity is established through serial clinical examination, serial radiographs, and advanced imaging. High-resolution computed tomography (CT) scan or cone beam computed tomography (CBCT) defines condylar morphology and excludes neoplasm; MRI assesses disc position and joint degeneration. Bone scintigraphy with single-photon emission computed tomography (SPECT) estimates relative metabolic activity—relative condylar uptake greater than ~55% suggests active

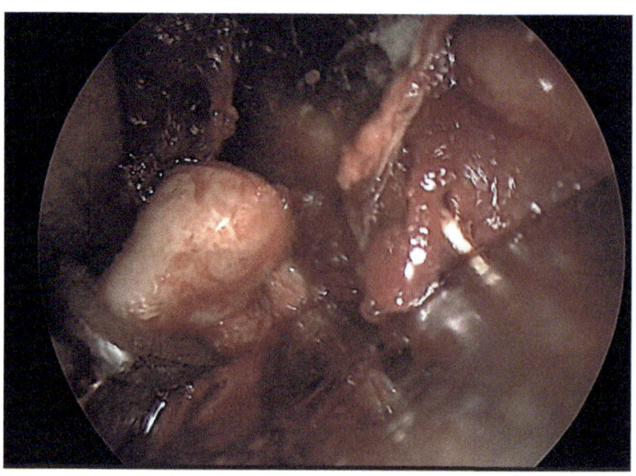

Fig. 2 Intraoral access to a proportional right TMJ condylectomy using endoscopic assistance and bone-borne surgical guides.

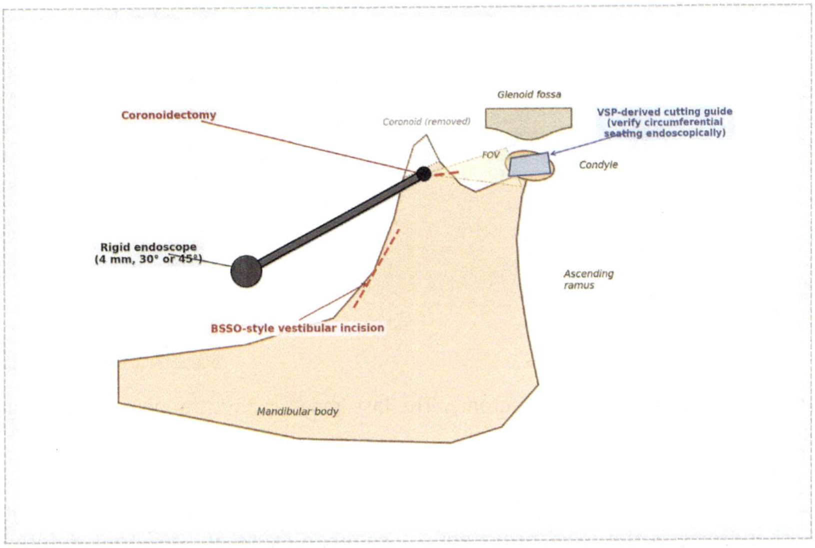

Fig. 3 Endoscopic-assisted intraoral approach. A BSSO-style vestibular incision exposes the lateral ramus and coronoid; the coronoid is removed, and the resulting window provides a direct corridor for endoscopically assisted access to the condyle.

growth, whereas equivocal findings (50%–55%) are not, by themselves, an indication for resection and warrant serial examination with repeat imaging at 6 to 12 months until progression is documented (algorithm 1) (Fig. 4).[4] VSP is the default planning modality; 3-dimensional simulation defines osteotomy orientation and volume, predicts mandibular autorotation and occlusal change, and generates patient-specific cutting guides (Figs. 5 and 1).

Condylectomy

Two variants address active CH. High condylectomy removes the superior 3 to 5 mm of the condylar head, including the presumed hyperactive growth center, and typically requires a secondary orthognathic procedure to correct residual asymmetry.[5,6] Proportional condylectomy removes a VSP-defined wedge calculated to restore symmetric condylar height in a single stage, preserving sufficient height for joint stability and occlusal normalization (Fig. 6). In either variant, the osteotomy is oriented perpendicular to the long axis of the condylar neck; a malleable retractor is placed medial to the neck before the saw; the lateral pterygoid is released if indicated; and a viable disc is preserved whenever possible. Temporary occlusal guidance before closure confirms midline alignment and cant reduction—the single most reliable safeguard against residual asymmetry. Either corridor described above may be used.

In correctly selected patients, condylectomy stabilizes mandibular growth and improves symmetry, and recurrence is uncommon when biologic activity has been accurately identified.[5,6] Reported complications include transient facial nerve weakness, occlusal instability, and persistent asymmetry from incomplete resection.

Pearl: The objective is not to *shorten* the condyle but to eliminate the active growth center while preserving joint function; planning must account for how mandibular autorotation will affect the posterior occlusion.

Pitfall: Under-resection is more common than over-resection and is the usual cause of persistent deviation or the need for secondary surgery.

Benign neoplasms of the temporomandibular joint

Benign tumors of the mandibular condyle are uncommon but represent the most frequent neoplastic processes requiring TMJ resection.[7] The central question is not simply tumor

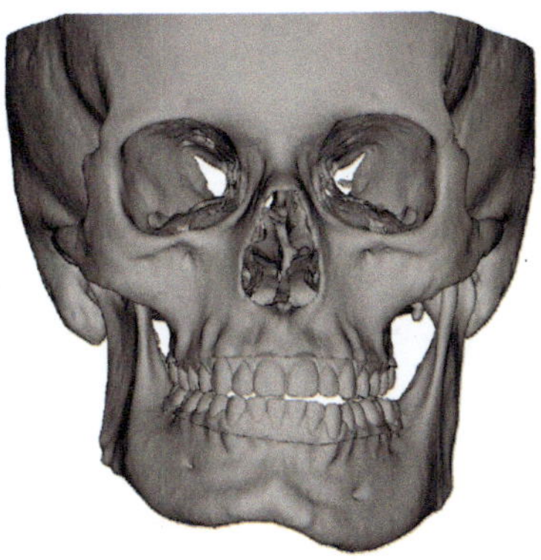

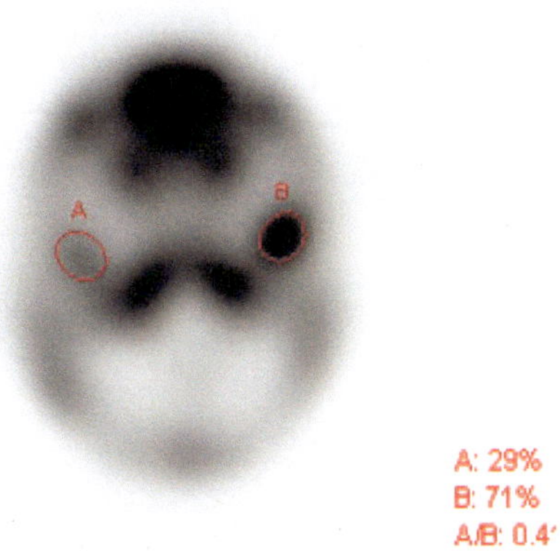

Fig. 4 Image on the left is a 3-dimensional reconstruction of a CT of the facial bones showing mandibular asymmetry and a left posterior open bite, consistent with left condylar pathology versus hyperplasia. The image on the right showcases a SPECT-CT with evidence of increased growth activity in the left condyle (71% compared to 29%).

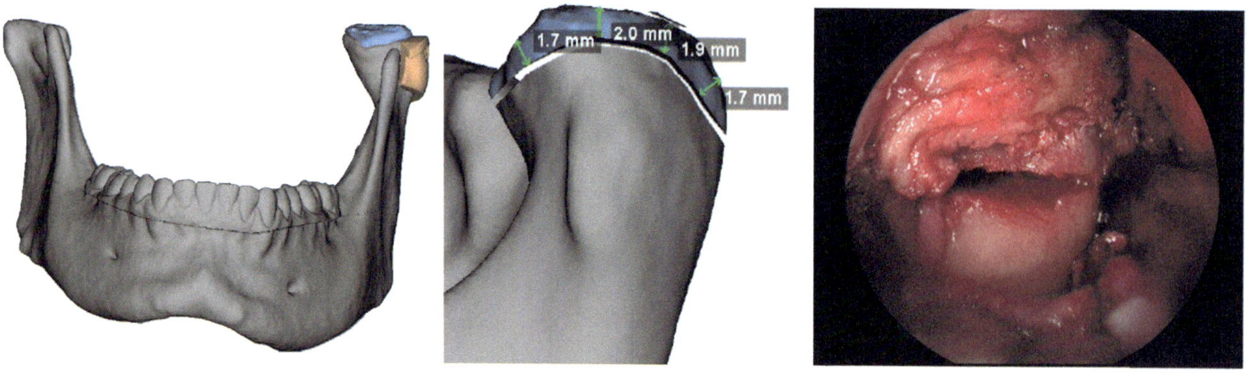

Fig. 5 VSP session demonstrating the projected condylectomy. The last image is an intraoperative photograph of the completed condylectomy cut, before delivery of the specimen.

removal but preservation—or restoration—of joint function and occlusal stability. Osteochondroma is the most prevalent lesion; a group of synovial, crystalline, and proliferative lesions accounts for most of the remainder.

Osteochondroma

Osteochondroma typically presents with progressive facial asymmetry, mandibular deviation, occlusal cant, and a contralateral posterior open bite.[8] Unlike the diffuse overgrowth of hyperplasia, it is a focal exophytic lesion arising from the condylar head, characterized radiographically by continuity of cortical and medullary bone with the underlying condyle. High-resolution CBCT defines lesion extent and its relationship to the glenoid fossa; MRI evaluates disc displacement and joint integrity.[9]

The operative objective is complete excision while preserving uninvolved joint structures, with resection level dictated by structural involvement of the condylar head rather than tumor size (algorithm 2).[10] Small pedunculated lesions with a preserved condyle are managed by local excision and contouring; sessile lesions involving part of the head with a preserved neck are treated by proportional condylectomy with a VSP wedge; extensive lesions that destroy the head or extend into the neck require complete condylectomy with immediate reconstruction. Recurrence after complete excision is rare; incomplete resection of the cartilaginous cap is the most common cause of persistent deformity.[8]

Pearl: The choice among local excision, proportional condylectomy, and complete condylectomy should be based on structural involvement of the condylar head, not tumor size alone.

Synovial, crystalline, and proliferative lesions

A group of benign intra-articular lesions shares overlapping clinical and radiographic features—joint swelling, pain, crepitus, and episodic locking—yet differs in biology and aggressiveness. Several are benign but locally aggressive and may erode the glenoid fossa and involve the skull base, a behavior that shifts management decisively. Arthroscopy plays a dual role: it secures a tissue diagnosis under direct vision and, in limited disease, can be therapeutic, while aggressive or skull base disease is treated by open arthroplasty and, when joint architecture is destroyed, by total joint replacement.

Synovial chondromatosis is a proliferative synovial disorder in which metaplastic cartilaginous nodules form within the joint and detach as loose bodies; imaging demonstrates multiple loose bodies or calcified nodules within the joint space.[11,12] (Fig. 7).

Chondrocalcinosis (calcium pyrophosphate deposition disease, or pseudogout) is a crystal deposition arthropathy in

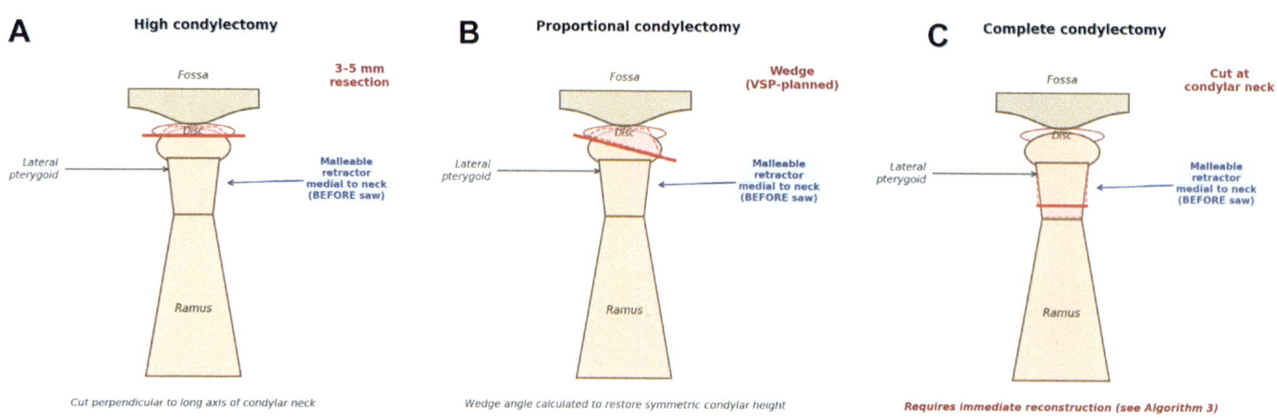

Fig. 6 Osteotomy orientation for condylectomy variants. (*A*) High condylectomy removes the superior 3 to 5 mm perpendicular to the long axis of the condylar neck. (*B*) Proportional condylectomy removes a VSP-planned wedge to restore symmetric condylar height. (*C*) Complete condylectomy is performed at the neck and requires immediate reconstruction. In all variants, a retractor is positioned medial to the neck before the saw.

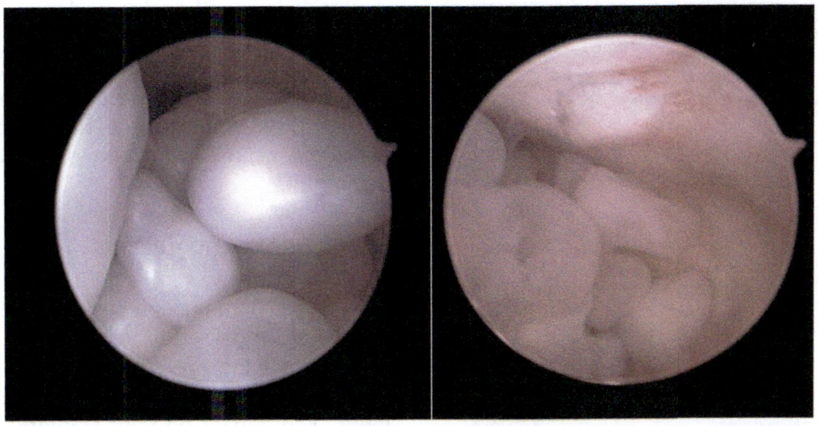

Fig. 7 Arthroscopic images of biopsy-proven synovial chondromatosis. Note the cartilaginous nodules floating in the joint space.

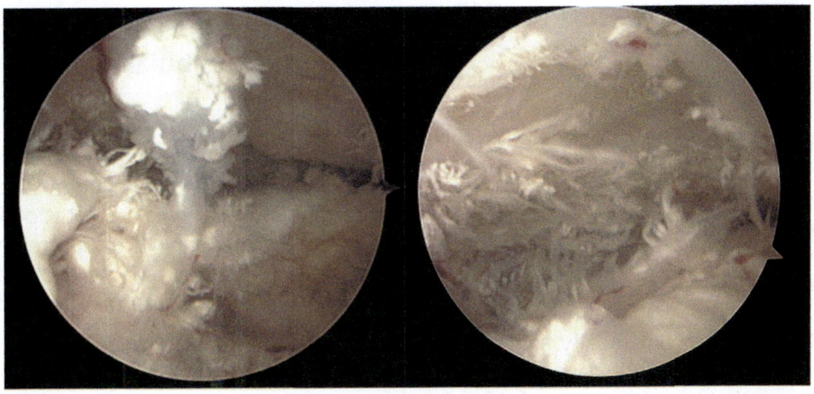

Fig. 8 Arthroscopic images showing biopsy-proven calcium pyrophosphate deposition, consistent with pseudogout.

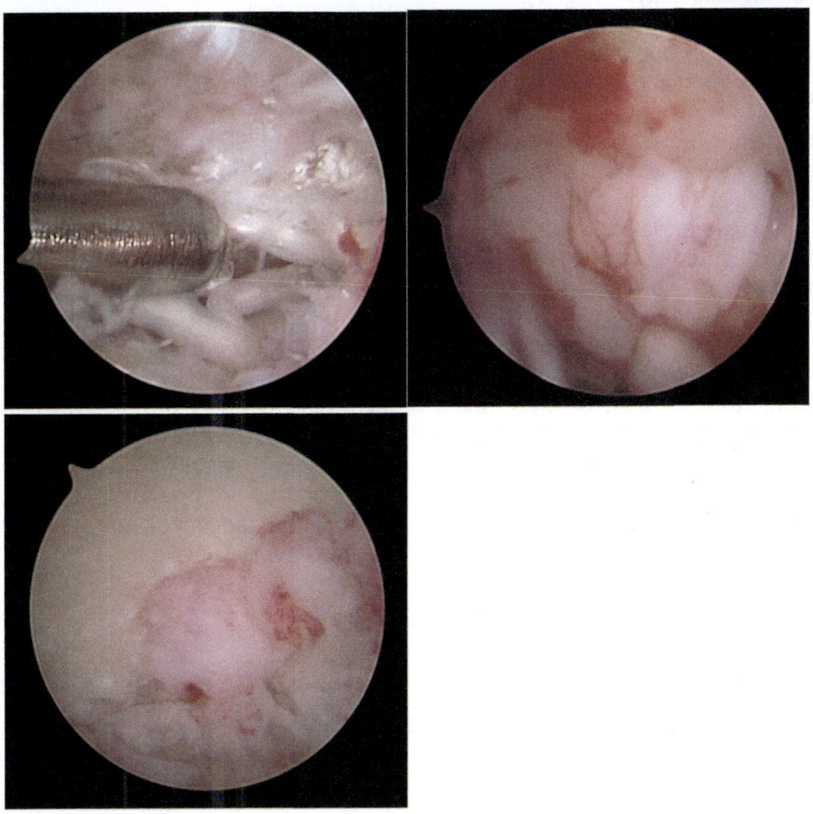

Fig. 9 Arthroscopic images of biopsy-proven CCMN. Note the similarity of the pathology to pseudogout, with crystal deposition noted in the first image. The third image showcases the beginning of skull base violation along the glenoid fossa, which highlights the locally aggressive nature of the disease process.

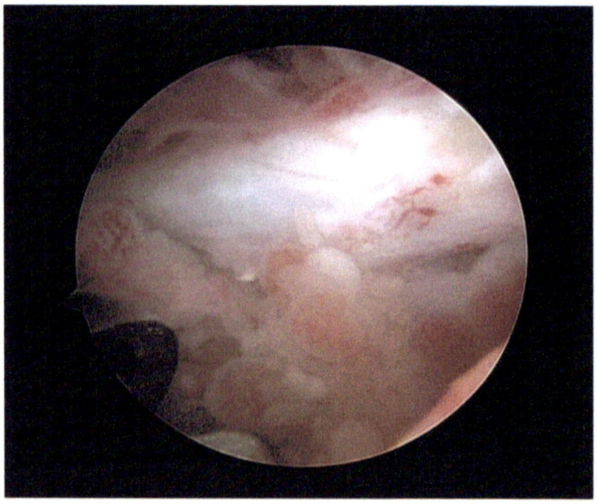

Fig. 10 Arthroscopic images of a case of biopsy-proven PVNS.

which calcified intra-articular masses may mimic neoplasm radiographically. Indolent crystal deposition without progressive joint destruction may be managed by debridement followed by in-office steroid injections and observation.[13] (Fig. 8).

Calcified chondroid mesenchymal neoplasm (CCMN) is a recently characterized entity—distinct from both synovial chondromatosis and chondrocalcinosis—defined by a chondroid matrix with calcification and recurrent FN1 and FGFR1/FGFR2 gene fusions.[14] In the TMJ it is benign but locally aggressive, with a propensity for bony erosion and skull base extension. The term has at times been applied loosely to crystal-deposition disease, but CCMN represents a separate neoplastic process and should be diagnosed histologically.[14] (Fig. 9).

Pigmented villonodular synovitis (PVNS; diffuse-type tenosynovial giant cell tumor) is a benign but locally destructive proliferation of synovium containing hemosiderin, characteristically low in signal on T1-and T2-weighted MRI.[15] Like CCMN, it can erode the fossa and extend toward the skull base, and recurrence is common after incomplete synovectomy (Fig. 10).

Operative selection is between arthroscopic and open management (Algorithm 2). Arthroscopic loose-body removal with synovectomy is appropriate for limited disease without joint expansion or skull base involvement and offers symptomatic relief with low morbidity; it also yields the diagnostic specimen that directs definitive treatment.[1,16] Open arthroplasty with thorough synovectomy is preferred for extensive disease, large loose bodies, joint expansion, fossa erosion, or after failed arthroscopy. When a locally aggressive lesion—particularly CCMN or PVNS—has destroyed condylar architecture or involves the skull base, management escalates to total joint replacement, frequently after the diagnosis has first been established arthroscopically (see Figs. 9 and 10).[17]

Pearl: In proliferative and crystalline disease the goal is removal of loose bodies, complete synovectomy, and relief of mechanical obstruction—not radical resection. Skull base involvement or aggressive erosion, as may occur with CCMN or PVNS, shifts management toward open resection and joint replacement; recurrence is most common when synovectomy is incomplete.

Other benign neoplasms

Many other benign condylar lesions are too rare for individual discussion; representative entities and their general management principles are summarized in Table 1. Management is dictated by histopathologic diagnosis, extent of bony involvement, and impact on joint stability; when significant condylar destruction is present, reconstruction follows the principles used in oncologic resection.[18]

Malignant lesions involving the temporomandibular joint

Primary malignant tumors of the TMJ are rare; when they occur they most often arise from the condyle, adjacent ramus, or skull base and include chondrosarcoma, osteosarcoma, and synovial sarcoma, with metastatic disease less common.[19] Patients may present with progressive pain, swelling, rapid asymmetry, trismus, or paresthesia, and imaging typically demonstrates ill-defined margins and cortical erosion.[20]

Preoperative evaluation

A comprehensive oncologic workup is mandatory. Contrast-enhanced CT and gadolinium MRI define the extent of bony and soft-tissue involvement, including extension to the fossa or skull base; PET-CT assists staging and identification of metastatic disease. Tissue diagnosis is obtained by image-guided biopsy, and the biopsy tract is positioned so that it can be excised en bloc with the specimen. Multidisciplinary planning with head and neck oncology, radiation oncology, and reconstructive surgery is essential.

Oncologic resection

The objective is complete en bloc resection with negative margins; piecemeal excision is contraindicated.[19] Isolated condylar disease may require complete condylectomy; ramus extension may necessitate segmental mandibulectomy with 1.5 to 2 cm of grossly normal bone; and fossa or skull base involvement requires composite resection, sometimes in collaboration with neurosurgery. Frozen-section analysis confirms margin adequacy, and reconstruction is not begun until margins are confirmed negative.

Table 1 Less common benign lesions of the temporomandibular joint and general management principles

Lesion	Typical presentation	Imaging	General management
Chondromyxoid fibroma	Localized pain or swelling	Lytic condylar lesion	En bloc excision with margin
Osteoma	Slow-growing mass	Dense radiopaque lesion	Local excision; observation if asymptomatic
Chondroblastoma	Painful swelling	Well-defined lytic lesion	Curettage or resection by aggressiveness
Central giant cell lesion	Expansile radiolucency	Multiloculated radiolucent defect	Curettage or segmental resection if aggressive

Algorithm 1. Condylar Hyperplasia: Workup and Selection of Resection

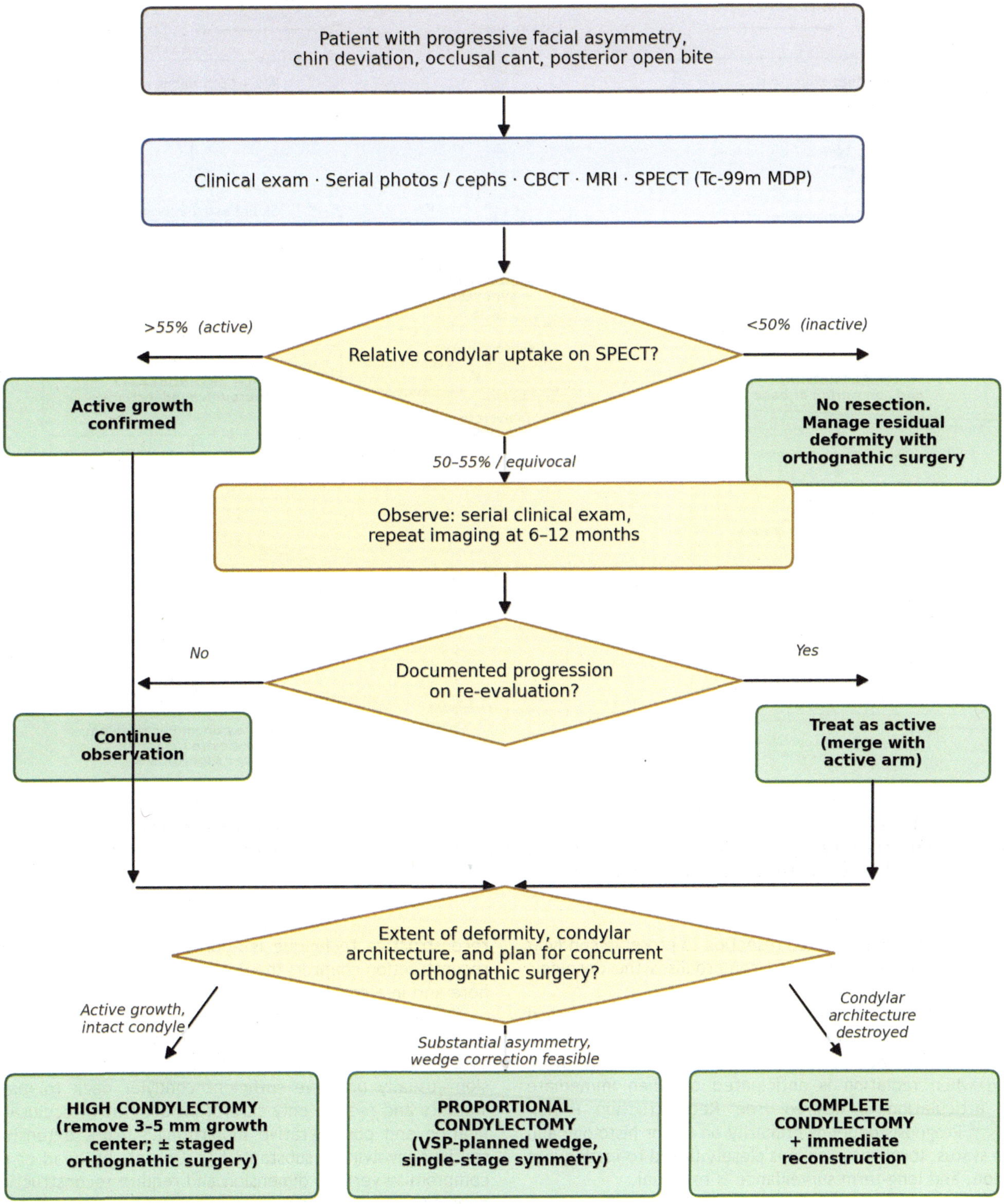

Across all arms: VSP-planned osteotomy · medial protection with malleable retractor before saw · intraoperative occlusal verification before closure.

Fig. 11 Algorithm 1—CH: workup and selection of resection variant, including the pathway for equivocal SPECT findings (50%–55% uptake: observe with serial imaging at 6–12 months before treating as active).

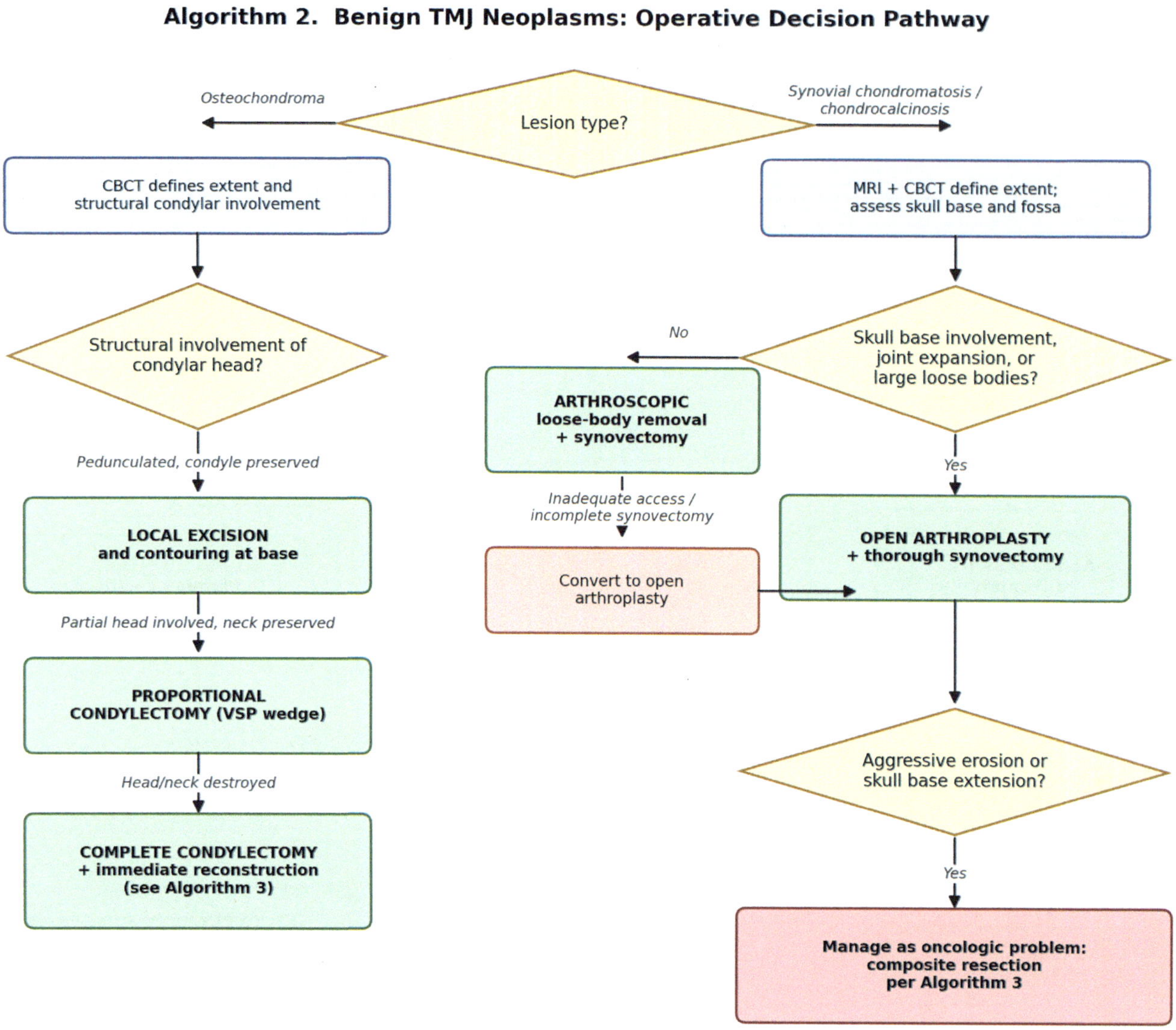

Fig. 12 Algorithm 2—Benign TMJ neoplasms: osteochondroma escalation (local excision → proportional → complete condylectomy) and arthroscopic-versus-open management of synovial, crystalline, and proliferative lesions, with escalation to open resection and joint replacement for skull base involvement or aggressive erosion.

Pitfall: Attempting a limited resection to preserve condylar height risks positive margins and compromises the oncologic outcome.

Reconstruction must restore mandibular continuity, vertical height, and articulation while accommodating potential adjuvant therapy; alloplastic total joint replacement is often favored when radiation is anticipated or when immediate stable articulation is desired (see Reconstruction Principles).[21,22] Prognosis depends primarily on tumor histology and margin status, local recurrence is closely linked to inadequate resection, and long-term surveillance is essential.

Reconstruction Principles after temporomandibular joint resection

Reconstruction is guided by defect size, patient age, and the biologic behavior of the underlying pathology; the goals—restoration of mandibular height, preservation of occlusion, and reestablishment of functional articulation—are consistent across hyperplasia, benign neoplasia, and malignancy. Detailed reconstructive technique is addressed in the dedicated TMJ reconstruction chapter; the decision framework is summarized here and in algorithm 3.

Not all resections require formal reconstruction. Limited superior and proportional resections—such as high condylectomy for hyperplasia or small osteochondroma excision—usually preserve sufficient condylar neck to maintain stability and require only careful intraoperative occlusal verification and postoperative monitoring.[23] More extensive resections involving a substantial portion of the head or ramus compromise vertical dimension and require reconstruction. In growing patients, costochondral grafting provides a biologic substitute with adaptive potential, though overgrowth and resorption must be anticipated.[24] Segmental defects are reliably restored with a vascularized free fibula, which also permits later dental rehabilitation. Patient-specific alloplastic total joint replacement offers predictable height and immediate stability and is favored in adults, after failed autogenous reconstruction, and when radiation is planned; composite oncologic defects are best managed by combined free fibula and alloplastic fossa and condyle.[21,25]

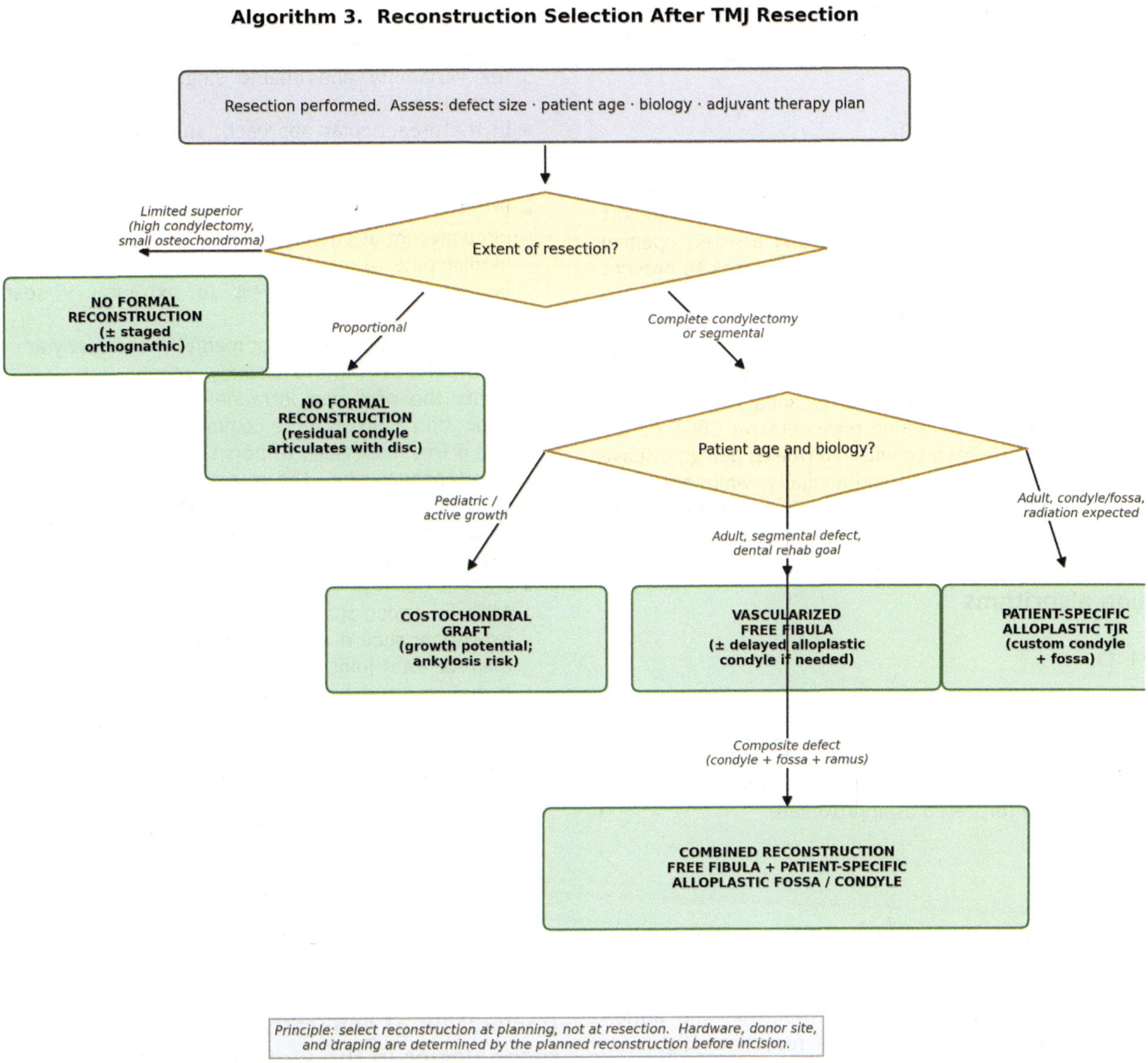

Fig. 13 Algorithm 3—Reconstruction selection after temporomandibular joint (TMJ) resection, matching reconstructive option to defect extent, patient age, biology, and adjuvant therapy plan.

Table 2 Representative outcomes after operative management of temporomandibular joint pathology

Procedure	Outcome	Recurrence/failure
High condylectomy (active CH)	Growth arrest in ~90% of correctly selected cases	Rare when biologic activity is correctly identified
Proportional condylectomy with VSP	Single-stage symmetric occlusion in selected cases	Undercorrection more common than over-correction
Osteochondroma resection	Symptomatic and esthetic improvement in most	Local recurrence rare with complete excision
Synovial/proliferative (arthroscopic)	Symptom relief in limited disease	Possible if synovectomy incomplete
Synovial/proliferative (open + TJR)	Durable relief in extensive or aggressive disease	Uncommon after complete synovectomy/replacement
Oncologic resection (margin-negative)	Local control linked to margin status	Recurrence linked to inadequate margins
Alloplastic TJR after resection	Predictable height and articulation; radiation-tolerant	Hardware complications uncommon

Pearl: The decision to reconstruct—and the choice of modality—is made at planning, based on anticipated postoperative mandibular stability, not at the time of resection.

Functional rehabilitation

Regardless of reconstructive modality, postoperative rehabilitation is critical. A liquid diet for 1 week is advanced to soft consistency over 4 to 6 weeks. Active and assisted opening exercises begin within the first postoperative week to prevent fibrosis and ankylosis; stacked tongue depressors or mouth-opening devices are introduced at 2 to 4 weeks and continued for 3 to 6 months toward an opening of at least 35 mm. Light vertical elastics guide a planned occlusal change, with orthodontic finishing coordinated when a secondary orthognathic component is planned. A baseline postoperative CBCT (or CT for oncologic cases) is obtained within 6 weeks; benign disease is followed at 6 and 12 months and annually, while oncologic surveillance follows the histology-specific multidisciplinary protocol.[24]

Decision algorithms

Figs. 11–13.

Clinical results

Representative outcomes are summarized in Table 2; reported ranges should be interpreted as approximate.

Summary

Pathologic conditions of the TMJ requiring resection are uncommon but demand disciplined judgment and early diagnosis. Treatment begins with distinguishing biologic behavior, defining the extent of structural involvement, and anticipating the functional consequences of resection. High condylectomy remains the cornerstone for active CH and selected benign lesions, with proportional condylectomy and VSP allowing single-stage symmetry, while complete excision is essential in osteochondroma. Proliferative, crystalline, and locally aggressive synovial lesions—including CCMN and PVNS—are frequently diagnosed arthroscopically and treated by synovectomy, or when joint architecture is destroyed or the skull base is involved, by open resection and total joint replacement. Malignant disease requires margin-negative en bloc resection over preservation of joint anatomy. Reconstruction is individualized and selected at the planning stage. Across all entities, the most common error is under-resection; durable outcomes depend on eliminating pathologic tissue, restoring occlusion, and instituting early functional rehabilitation.

Clinics care points

- Confirm biologic activity before resecting condylar hyperplasia: relative condylar SPECT uptake >55% supports active growth; equivocal findings (50–55%) warrant serial imaging at 6–12 months, not surgery.
- Use virtual surgical planning as the default for any condylectomy; VSP-derived guides reduce medial-cortex variability and enable single-stage proportional correction.
- In the preauricular approach, subperiosteal elevation on the lateral zygomatic arch is the principal facial-nerve protection maneuver.
- In the endoscopic-assisted intraoral approach, confirm circumferential cutting-guide seating — including the medial pole — under direct endoscopic visualization before osteotomy; convert to extraoral if seating cannot be confirmed.
- Place a malleable retractor medial to the condylar neck before the saw, in every condylectomy.
- Verify the occlusion intraoperatively before closure; under-correction is more common than over-correction and drives most cases of persistent deviation.
- In osteochondroma, the resection level is dictated by structural involvement of the condylar head, not by tumor size; incomplete excision of the cartilaginous cap is the leading cause of recurrence.
- Suspect CCMN or PVNS when a benign-appearing intra-articular lesion shows aggressive erosion or skull-base extension; secure an arthroscopic tissue diagnosis and plan for total joint replacement.
- In malignancy, perform complete en bloc resection with negative frozen-section margins before initiating reconstruction; piecemeal excision is contraindicated.
- Choose the reconstructive modality at planning, not at resection — costochondral graft in growing patients, vascularized fibula for segmental defects, alloplastic TJR in adults or when radiation is anticipated, and combined fibula plus alloplastic fossa-condyle for composite oncologic defects — and begin active opening exercises within the first postoperative week.

Declaration of generative AI and AI-assisted technologies in the writing process

During the preparation of this work, the authors used generative artificial intelligence tools (OpenAI ChatGPT and image-generation assistance) to create illustrations intended solely for educational visualization. All images were reviewed, edited, and verified by the authors. No AI-generated content was used to generate original research data, patient information, or diagnostic imaging. The authors take full responsibility for the accuracy, originality, and integrity of all text and figures included in this work.

References

1. McCain JP, Hossameldin RH. Advanced arthroscopy of the temporomandibular joint. Atlas Oral Maxillofac Surg Clin North Am 2011; 19:145–67.
2. Wolford LM, Movahed R, Perez DE. A classification system for conditions causing condylar hyperplasia. J Oral Maxillofac Surg 2014;72:567–95.
3. Wolford LM, Karras SC, Mehra P. Concomitant temporomandibular joint and orthognathic surgery: a preliminary report. J Oral Maxillofac Surg 2002;60:356–62.
4. Saridin CP, Raijmakers PG, Al Shamma S, et al. Comparison of planar bone scintigraphy and single photon emission computed

tomography in patients suspected of having unilateral condylar hyperactivity. Int J Oral Maxillofac Surg 2009;38:942–6.
5. Wolford LM, Mehra P, Reiche-Fischel O, et al. Efficacy of high condylectomy for management of condylar hyperplasia. Am J Orthod Dentofacial Orthop 2002;121:136–50.
6. Brusati R, Pedrazzoli M, Colletti G. Functional results after condylectomy in active laterognathism. J Craniomaxillofac Surg 2010; 38:179–84.
7. Carlson ER, Marx RE. The ameloblastoma: primary, curative surgical management. J Oral Maxillofac Surg 2006;64:484–94.
8. Ord RA, Warburton G, Caccamese JF. Osteochondroma of the condyle: review of 8 cases. Int J Oral Maxillofac Surg 2010;39:523–8.
9. Chen MJ, Yang C, Zhang SY, et al. Osteochondroma of the mandibular condyle: a classification system based on computed tomographic appearances. J Craniofac Surg 2014;25:1703–6.
10. Wolford LM, Mehra P, Franco P. Use of conservative condylectomy for treatment of osteochondroma of the mandibular condyle. J Oral Maxillofac Surg 2002;60:262–8.
11. Milgram JW. Synovial osteochondromatosis: a histopathological study of thirty cases. J Bone Joint Surg Am. 1977;59:792–801.
12. Holmlund AB, Eriksson L, Reinholt FP. Synovial chondromatosis of the temporomandibular joint: clinical, surgical and histopathological aspects. Int J Oral Maxillofac Surg 2003;32:143–7.
13. Choi DD, Smith DH, Davis C, et al. Arthroscopic diagnosis and medical management of calcium pyrophosphate deposition disease in the temporomandibular joint. Int J Oral Maxillofac Surg 2020;49: 1618–21.
14. Liu YJ, Wang W, Yeh J, et al. Calcified chondroid mesenchymal neoplasms with FN1–receptor tyrosine kinase gene fusions including FGFR2, FGFR1, MERTK, NTRK1, and TEK: a molecular and clinicopathologic analysis. Mod Pathol. 2021;34:1373–83.
15. Safaee M, Oh T, Sun MZ, et al. Pigmented villonodular synovitis of the temporomandibular joint with intracranial extension: a case series and systematic review. Head Neck 2015;37:1213–24.
16. Guarda-Nardini L, Piccotti F, Ferronato G, et al. Synovial chondromatosis of the temporomandibular joint: a case description with systematic literature review. Int J Oral Maxillofac Surg 2010; 39:745–55.
17. Vellutini EAS, Alonso N, Arap SS, et al. Functional reconstruction of temporomandibular joint after resection of pigmented villonodular synovitis with extension to infratemporal fossa and skull base: a case report. Surg J (N Y) 2016;2:e78–82.
18. Poveda-Roda R, Bagán JV, Sanchis JM, et al. Pseudotumors and tumors of the temporomandibular joint. A review. Med Oral Patol Oral Cir Bucal 2013;18:e392–402.
19. Schlieve T, McCoy JM, Carlson ER. Bone margin analysis for benign odontogenic tumors. Oral Maxillofac Surg Clin North Am 2017;29: 147–58.
20. Larheim TA, Abrahamsson AK, Kristensen M, et al. Temporomandibular joint diagnostics using CBCT. Dentomaxillofac Radiol 2015; 44:20140235.
21. Mercuri LG. Alloplastic temporomandibular joint replacement: rationale for the use of custom devices. Int J Oral Maxillofac Surg 2012;41:1033–40.
22. Warburton G, Mercuri LG. Alloplastic reconstruction of the temporomandibular joint in patients with dentofacial deformities. Atlas Oral Maxillofac Surg Clin North Am 2022;30:153–60.
23. Sidebottom AJ, Gruber E. One-year prospective outcome analysis and complications following total replacement of the temporomandibular joint with the TMJ Concepts system. Br J Oral Maxillofac Surg 2013;51:620–4.
24. Kaban LB, Bouchard C, Troulis MJ. A protocol for management of temporomandibular joint ankylosis in children. J Oral Maxillofac Surg 2009;67:1966–78.
25. Bocchialini G, Castellani A, Negrini S, et al. Total joint replacement for immediate reconstruction following ablative surgery for primary tumors of the temporomandibular joint. J Pers Med 2023; 13:1021.

Combined Temporomandibular Joint and Orthognathic Reconstruction

Briana J. Burris, DDS [a,b,*], Jeffrey Hajibandeh, DDS, MD [b,c], Julian Wilson, DDS [d]

KEYWORDS

• TMJ arthropathy • TMJ arthritis • Reconstruction • Dentofacial anomaly • Orthognathic surgery • Total alloplastic joint replacement

KEY POINTS

- Comorbid temporomandibular joint (TMJ) arthropathies and dentofacial anomalies pose complex diagnostic and treatment planning dilemmas.
- Surgical goals of combined reconstruction include: symptomatic and functional relief of an end-stage TMJ arthropathy, functional occlusion, and esthetic facial harmony.
- Simultaneous correction of concomitant TMJ arthropathies and dentofacial anomalies requires diligent presurgical sequencing and planning, to achieve planned surgical movements.
- Planned surgical movements are limited by the patient's soft tissue envelope and must consider the arc of rotation necessary for mandibular opening.
- Use of patient-specific TMJ alloplasts requires precision during alignment and fixation, as intraoperative modifications are not possible. Orthognathic movements may need to be altered, requiring intraoperative hand-bending of stock hardware.

Introduction: Nature of the problem

Patients may present with unilateral or bilateral temporomandibular joint (TMJ) arthropathies and concomitant dentofacial anomalies, severely impacting: mastication, speech, respiration, and deglutination.[1] TMJ arthropathies are characterized by mandibular dysfunction (ie, hypomobility, hypermobility, and instability) and may or may not present with pain.[2]

Patients typically present in 1 of 3 ways

1. Patient presents with predominant chief complaint of a TMJ arthropathy, and is unaware of the impact of the co-existing dentofacial anomaly.
2. Patient presents with predominant chief complaint of a dentofacial anomaly with dental malocclusion and is unaware or asymptomatic at degenerated TMJ.
3. Patient is symptomatic at dysfunctional TMJ and is aware and bothered by coexisting dentofacial anomaly with malocclusion.

[a] Oral and Maxillofacial Residency Training Program, Massachusetts General Hospital, Boston, MA, USA
[b] Harvard Medical School and Harvard School of Dental Medicine, Boston, MA, USA
[c] Oral & Maxillofacial Surgery, Oral Medicine, & Dentistry, Massachusetts General Hospital, Boston, MA, USA
[d] University of California and Harbor-UCLA Medical Center, Los Angeles, CA, USA
* Corresponding author. 55 Fruit Street, Warren Building #1201, Boston, MA 02114.
E-mail address: bburris@mgh.harvard.edu

Patient education and understanding of the complexities associated with concomitant TMJ arthropathies and dentofacial anomalies with malocclusion is paramount, as extensive surgical reconstruction, including TMJ total alloplastic joint replacement (TJR) with simultaneous orthognathic surgery, may be indicated in effort to achieve asymptomatic, stable functional mandibular movements that end in repeatable, balanced occlusion.[2,3]

Surgical technique

Preoperative planning

- Initial questions to consider in patients planned for combined TJR and orthognathic surgery. The following questions determine subsequent presurgical timeline and surgical planning sequence:
  - Is a unilateral or bilateral TJR indicated?
    - If unilateral, a contralateral sagittal split osteotomy (vs vertical ramus osteotomy) may be indicated.
  - Is a single-stage or 2-stage TJR planned?
    - Single-stage TJR is defined as simultaneous condylectomy, fossa osteoplasty, and insertion of TJR prostheses
    - Two-stage TJR refers to 2 separate procedures:
      - Gap arthroplasty, including condylectomy, is performed. Obtain postprocedural CT (or cone-beam computed tomography [CBCT]) to be used for fabrication of TMJ prostheses
      - More than 3 months later: Return to operating room for necessary osteoplasty and insertion of TJR prostheses performed

Atlas Oral Maxillofacial Surg Clin N Am 34 (2026) 259-267

https://doi.org/10.1016/j.cxom.2026.05.007

Abbreviations

IOS	intraoral scan
PSI	patient-specific implant
TJR	total alloplastic joint replacement
TMJ	temporomandibular joint
TMJA-DFAM	TMJ arthropathies and dentofacial anomalies with malocclusion

- If 2-stage, open arthroplasty and condylectomy completion date will determine timeline for obtaining final CT scan to be used for fabrication of alloplast(s).
- Are presurgical orthodontic movements ongoing?
  - When is the anticipated end to active presurgical movements?
  - Recommend orthodontic-latency of ~4–6 weeks before obtaining CT and intraoral scan (IOS) to be used for fabrication of alloplast(s).

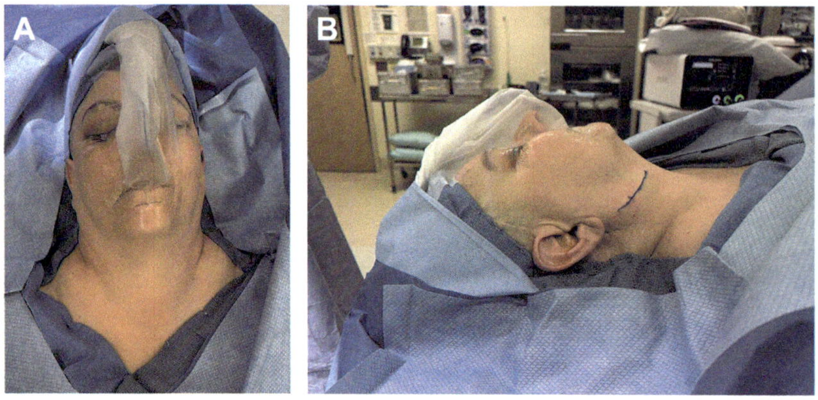

Fig. 1 (*A, B*) Photo of prepped and draped patient. Note the adhesive seal over nose and mouth.

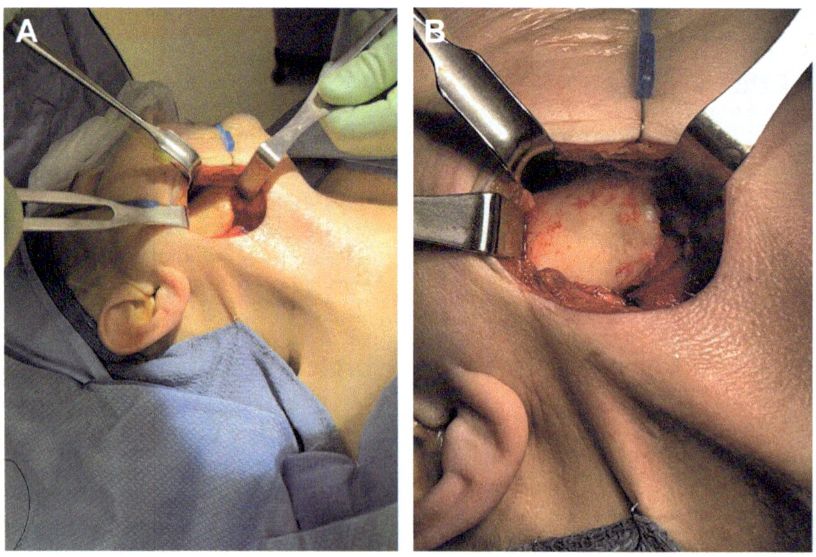

Fig. 2 (*A*) Modified submandibular exposure. (*B*) Closer view of right ramus exposure via submandibular incision.

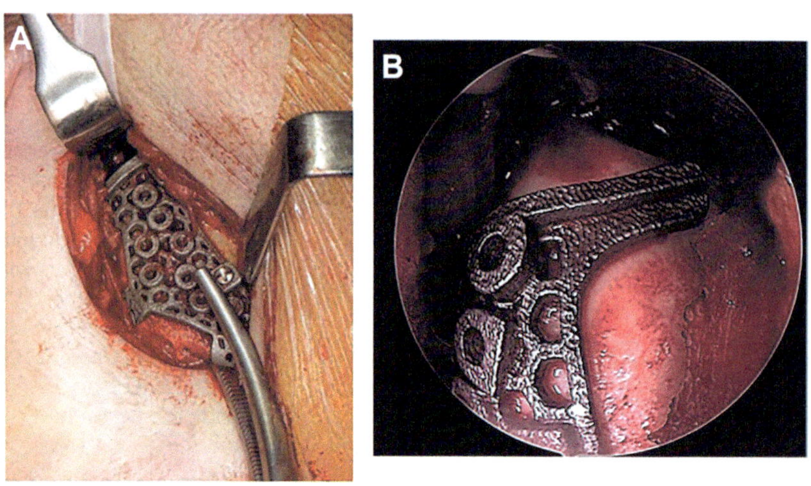

Fig. 3 (*A*) External view of cutting and fixation guide, sitting flush along the entire lateral aspect of the mandibular ramus (*B*) Endoscopic confirmation of adequate adaptation of the right condylar cutting and fixation guide, at the level of the sigmoid notch.

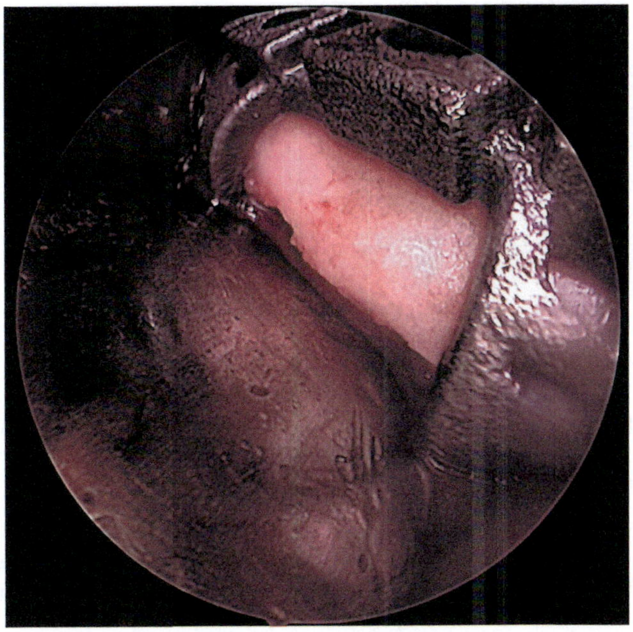

Fig. 4 Visual confirmation of appropriate adaptation of condylar cutting guide along the right mandibular angle.

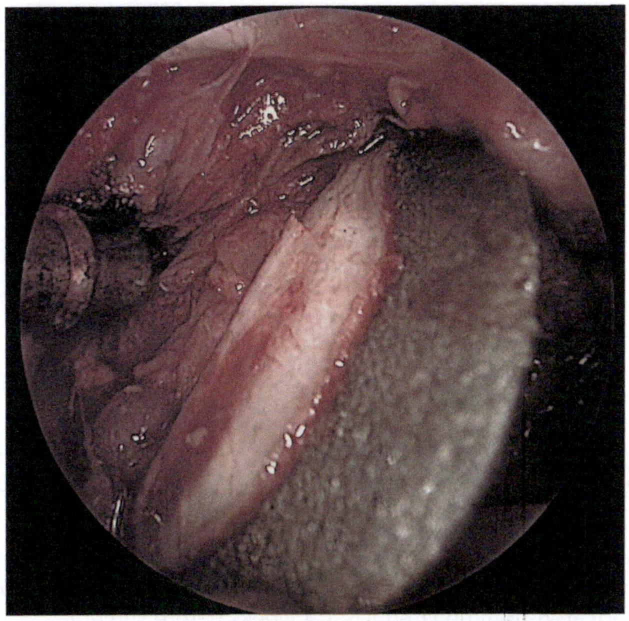

Fig. 6 Visual confirmation of completion of planned condylectomy, relative to the fixated cutting guide, reducing the height of the native mandibular ramus to the planned vertical height.

Presurgical virtual surgical planning of both the TJR and orthognathic movements will be completed at the same time.[3–6] When planning bilateral TMJ TJR, planning starts in the maxilla, achieving the ideal, optimized maxillary position before establishing occlusion. The mandibular prostheses' positions are determined by the maxillary position and occlusion.

Manufacturer's lead time for fabrication of the TMJ alloplast(s) determine surgical scheduling. Contemporary lead

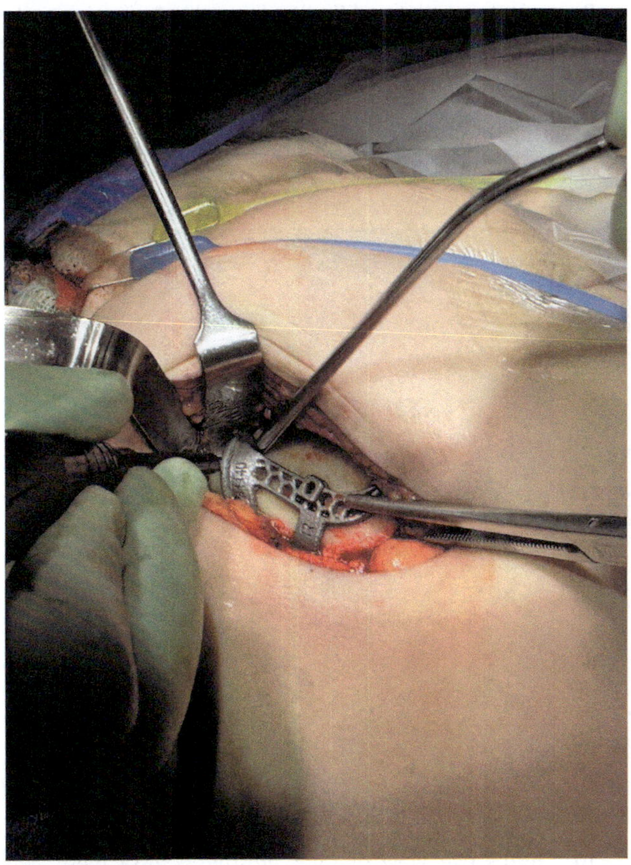

Fig. 5 Placement of condylectomy cutting guide via modified submandibular incision.

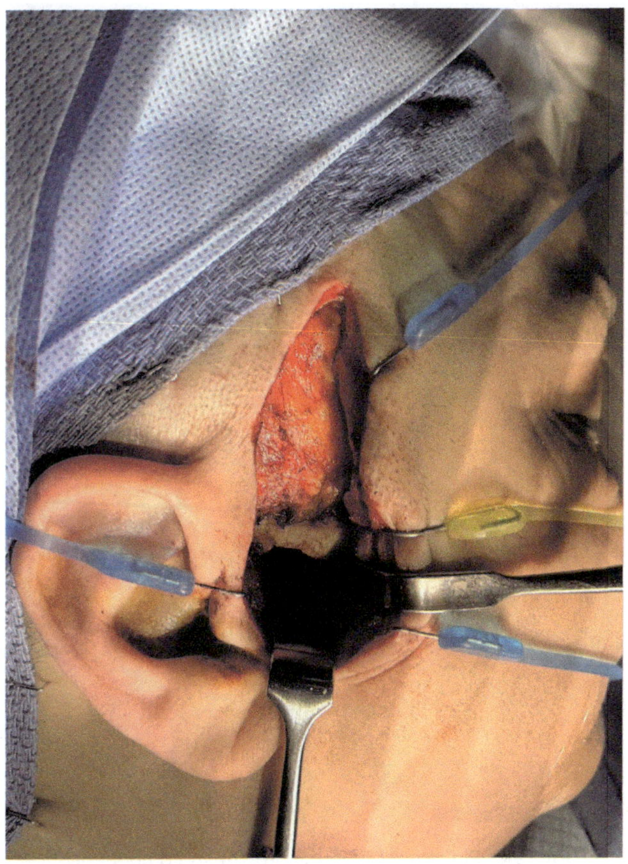

Fig. 7 Access through preauricular incision.

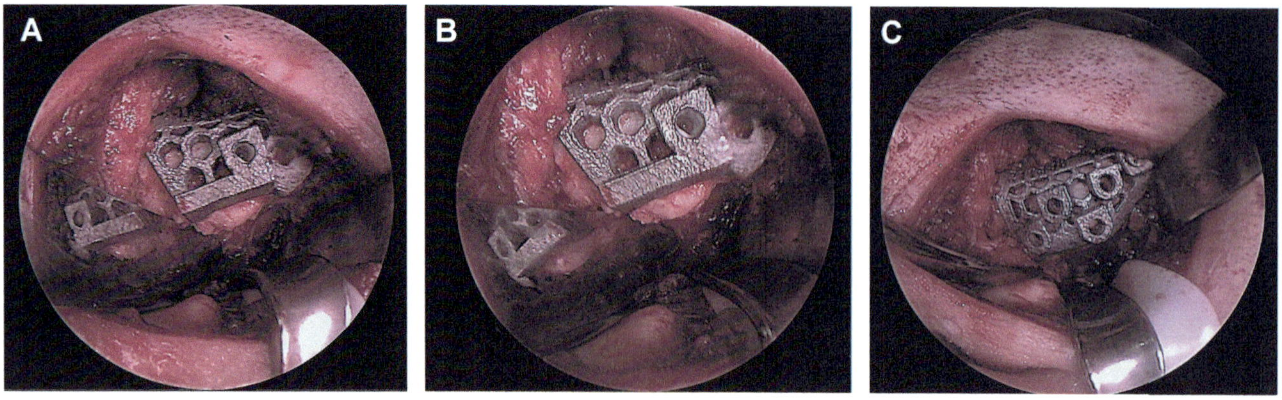

Fig. 8 (*A*) View of the right fossa reduction guide in place, flat edge of titanium guide indicates need for bony reduction of prominent articular eminence. (*B*) Closer view of the right fossa reduction guide in place, flat edge of titanium guide indicates need for bony reduction of prominent articular eminence. (*C*) Interval bony reduction completed, to allow for seating of the right fossa prosthesis.

time is 12–16 weeks. Patient-specific implants (PSIs) for Le Fort and/or genioplasty have a shorter lead time and can be fabricated from updated IOS 3–4 weeks before surgery.

Prep and patient positioning

- The TJR component of the procedure is sterile and should follow aseptic technique
  - Recommend use of adhesive coverings and drapes to seal off the oral cavity.
  - Prep with betadine, emphasis to cleaning external auditory canal

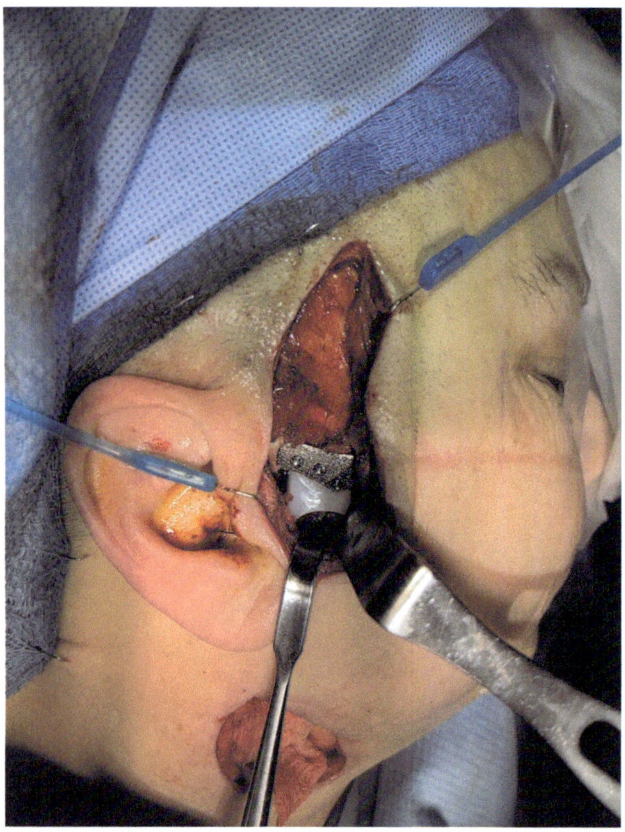

Fig. 9 Placement of fossa prosthesis component.

  - While the preauricular and submandibular incisions are open: any time the oral cavity is accessed, a sterile drape should be placed on top of all sterile instruments, and effort should be made to prevent saliva from contaminating the extraoral incisions.
- The orthognathic component of the procedure is clean contaminated
  - Prep of the oral cavity with betadine and/or chlorohexidine are recommended.

Surgical approach

- Preauricular and (modified) submandibular incisions are recommended for adequate access for insertion and fixation of glenoid fossa alloplast and the condylar component of the alloplast
  - Surgeon-dependent preference on which incision to perform first

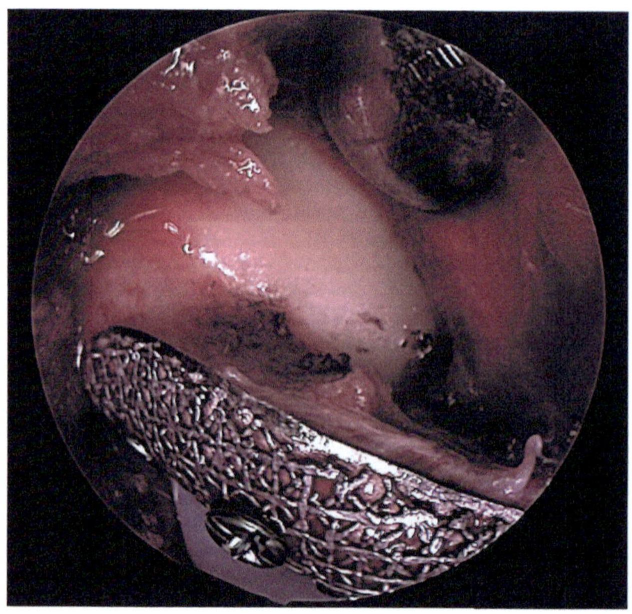

Fig. 10 Bird's eye view of right prosthetic fossa mesh, with appropriate adaptation along superior edge of the root of the zygoma.

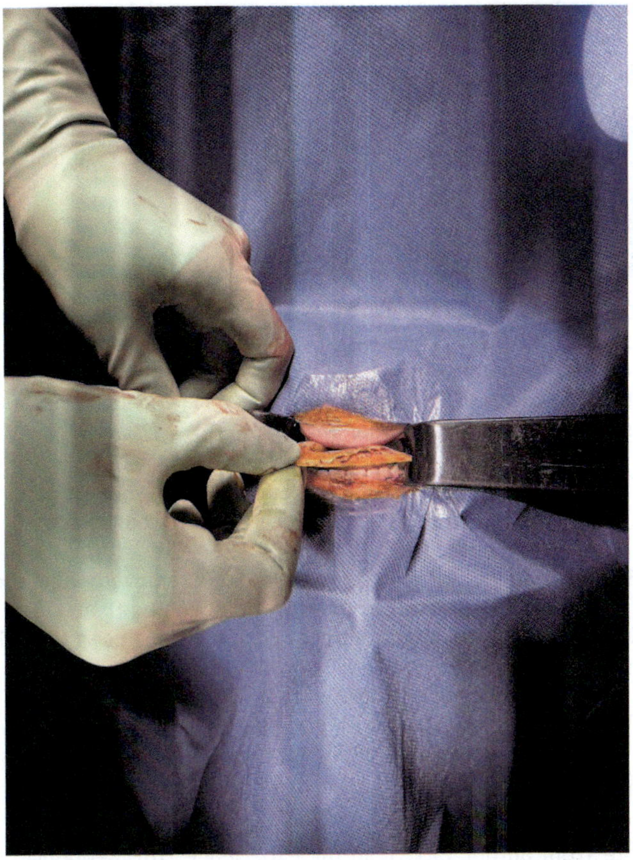

Fig. 11 Placement of oversheet drape for contaminated portion of procedure. Placement of occlusal guide before insertion and fixation of condylar prosthesis components.

  - Surgeon-dependent selection of modifications to preauricular incision, including endaural incision, temporal extension, and modified endaural (*invisicion*)
- Traditional vestibular incisions are used to access the maxilla, mandible, and genial region.
  - Care is taken to avoid subperiosteal dissection that directly communicates with the TMJ alloplast(s).

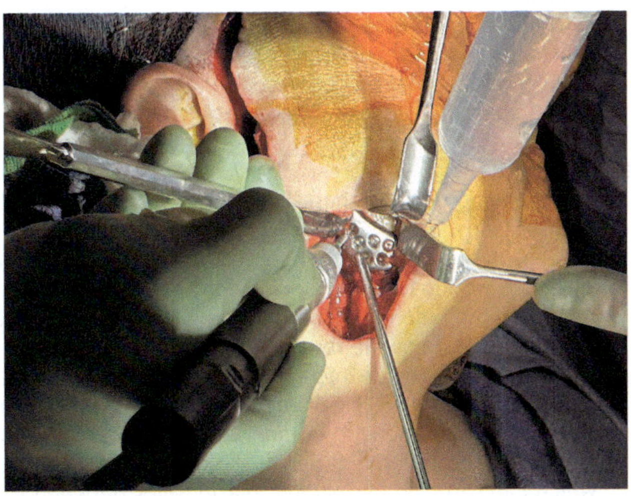

Fig. 12 Fixation of condylar prosthesis through modified submandibular incision.

Surgical procedure steps listed

Surgical steps for bilateral temporomandibular joint total joint replacement and Le Fort osteotomy ± genioplasty

1. Prepping and sterile draping is performed, isolating the field. See Fig. 1A, B.
2. The selected preauricular incision (or modification) and submandibular incisions are marked.
3. Administration of dilute epinephrine subcuticularly to help with hemostasis and hydro-dissection.
4. See Clayton M Davis's article, "Autogenous and Alloplastic Reconstruction of the Temporomandibular Joint," in this issue.
   a. Completion of condylectomies, fossa osteoplasty, coronoidectomies, and fixation of glenoid fossa prosthesis components. See Figs. 2–15.
5. The surgeon may elect to close the extraoral incisions before intraoral access for the Le Fort osteotomy.
   a. If preauricular and submandibular incisions are completely closed, recommend dressing wounds with cotton pads and clear adhesive bandages, before initiation of clean-contaminated, orthognathic component of surgery.
   b. If surgeon has concern for incorrect position of the TMJ prostheses and would like to defer wound closure until after orthognathic components:
      i. Pack the extraoral wounds with a wet laparotomy sponges and cover with 3M Ioban antimicrobial incise dressings
6. Traditional vestibular approach for maxillary exposure, including elevation of nasal floor.
7. Patient-specific positioning guides are fixated and should fit passively. See Fig. 15.
   a. Placement of patients in maxillomandibular fixation (MMF) may help confirm positioning of PSI.
8. Fixation of PSI or hand-bending of fixation plates
9. If discrepancy present between planned and actual hardware adaptation, low threshold to use occlusal splint; place patient in MMF and hand-bend fixation plates.
10. Perform genioplasty
11. Closure of intraoral wounds
    a. Sterile drape placed before incising Ioban drape to access extraoral wounds for reassessment of prosthesis position and wound closure

Surgical steps for unilateral temporomandibular joint total joint replacement, contralateral sagittal split osteotomy, and Le Fort osteotomy

1. For unilateral TMJ total joint replacement performed concurrently with a sagittal split osteotomy, the operative sequencing aims to minimize re-draping and transitions between clean and contaminated fields.
2. Begin on the TJR side in a sterile field, performing:
   a. Preauricular dissection
   b. Condylectomy (without surgical guide)
   c. Myofascial release of coronoid process
      i. Alternative: perform coronoidectomy
   d. Submandibular neck dissection with exposure of the mandibular ramus

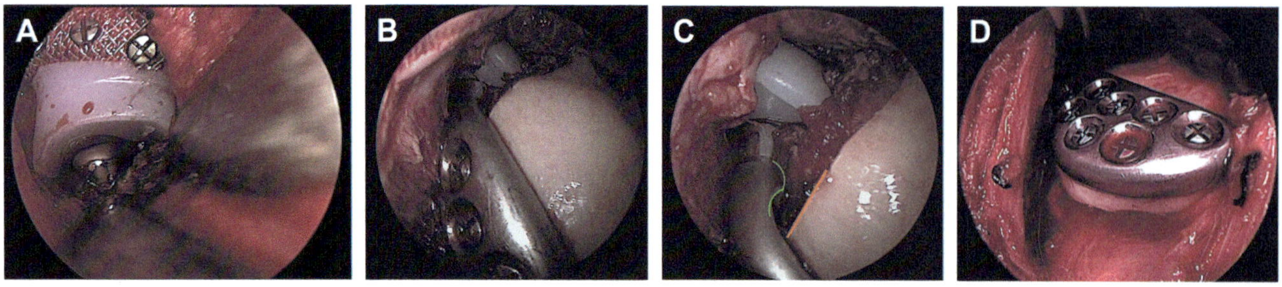

Fig. 13 (*A*) Confirmation of posterior-superior and medial position of the right prosthetic condylar head. (*B*) Confirmation of superior, posterior, and medial position of the right prosthetic condylar head relative to the prosthetic fossa. (*C*) Note the standard medial-curvature and projection of the prosthetic-condylar- neck (green *line*). If condylar osteotomy is not sufficiently inferior to the curvature (orange *line*), the condylar component can be laterally displaced, and will not be able to sit flush against the lateral mandibular ramus. (*D*) Visual confirmation of planned adaptation of patient-fitted condylar prosthesis and right mandibular angle.

   i. If utilizing surgical guide for condylectomy, fixation of guide precedes condylectomy and coronoidectomy
3. The fossa component is placed and fixated in its final orientation
4. Both surgical sites (preauricular and neck) are then covered with a lap sponge, and the TMJ region is additionally isolated with 3M Ioban antimicrobial incise adhesive drapes.
5. Transition to the clean-contaminated oral cavity to perform the contralateral sagittal split osteotomy and segments are split.
6. The patient is placed into intermaxillary fixation, and the sagittal split osteotomy of the mandible is definitively fixated while maintaining occlusion.
7. Once mandibular fixation is complete, return to the TJR site, re-prep on top of the Ioban drape.
   a. Place a second sterile drape over all areas except the Ioban-covered joint.
8. The Ioban is incised, the lap sponge removed, and the condylar prosthesis component is placed and fixated.
9. Final irrigation and closure of both incisions used for TJR access.
   a. Remainder of the case is clean contaminated.
10. Return to mouth for Le Fort osteotomy and/or genioplasty, before closure of all intraoral mucosal wounds. See Figs. 16–18.

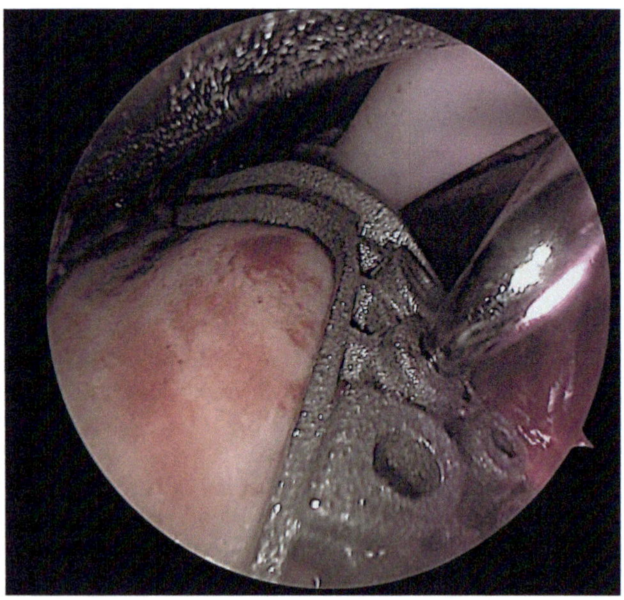

Fig. 14 Confirmation of adequate adaptation of the left condylar cutting and fixation guide, with guide sitting flush along the entire lateral aspect of the mandibular ramus. Tenacious masseter and temporalis muscles fibers along the superior ramus, in the region of the sigmoid notch, can result in inadequate adaptation of the cutting guide.

Note from author (J.W.): In my experience, this sequence is efficient and minimizes the need to completely re-drape while maintaining strict sterile-non-sterile separation.

Potential complications

Potential complications include standard complications from both TJR and orthognathic surgery.

- Hardware loosening and/or failure
- Infection
- Heterotopic bone formation
- Damage to adjacent structures
  - Facial nerve
  - Inferior alveolar nerve
  - Teeth, gums, lips, nasal structures
  - Middle ear structures
  - Middle cranial fossa structures
- Malocclusion
- Need for additional procedures
- Unanticipated or undesirable esthetic changes

Pearls and pitfalls

- Consider approaching these complex cases with 2 qualified surgeons.
  - Team approach (TJR-team vs orthognathic-team) can reduce workload for single surgeon
- Achieving the planned position of the patient-specific TJR alloplast is paramount for achieving accurate fit of patient-specific orthognathic hardware.
- TJR prostheses have significant rotational-variability of the condylar component within the glenoid fossa component. This allows for variation of the mandibular position, which can result in misleading relationships between the maxilla and mandible, especially before a planned Le Fort I osteotomy.

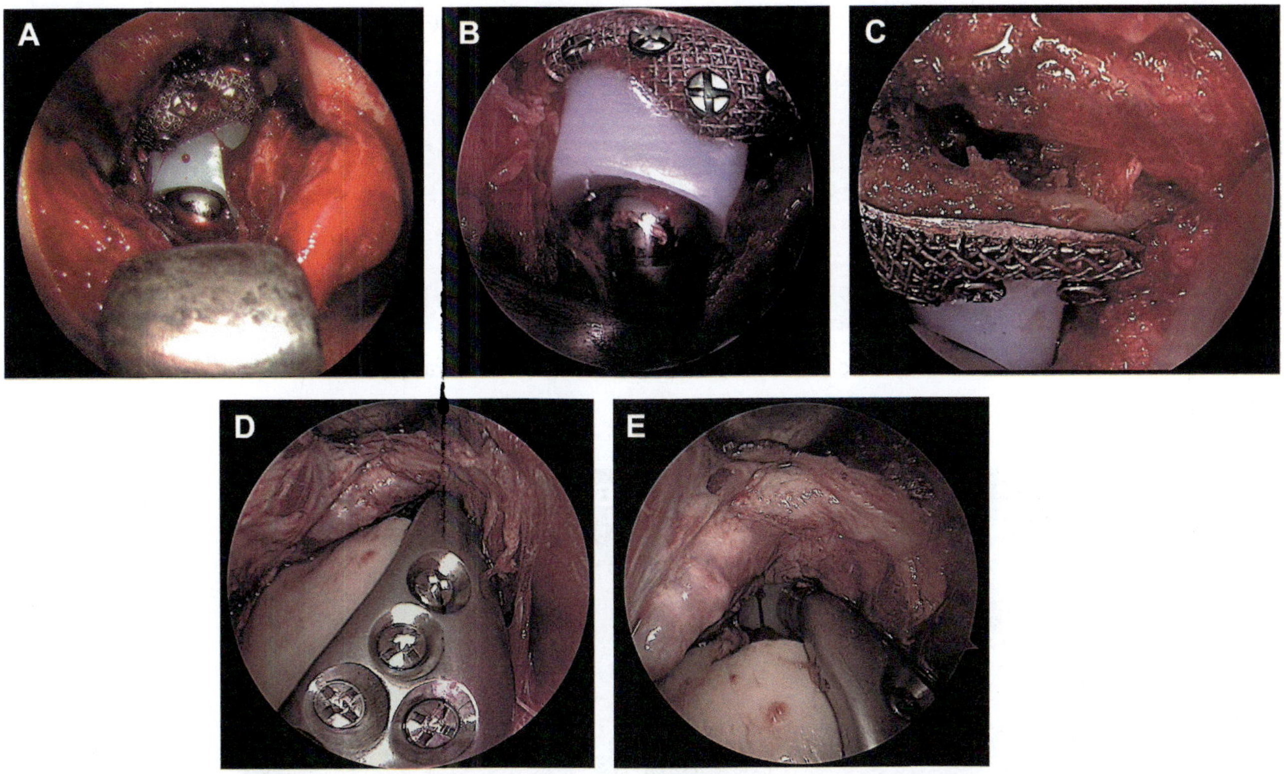

Fig. 15 (*A*) Confirmation of posterior-superior position of the left prosthetic condylar head. (*B*) Visual inspection from the pre-auricular incision to confirm superior, posterior, and medial position of the left prosthetic condylar head relative to the prosthetic fossa. (*C*) Bird's eye view of left prosthetic fossa mesh, with appropriate adaptation along superior edge of the root of the zygoma. (*D*) Confirmation of sufficient condylectomy allows for planned adaptation of the condylar prosthesis; without lateral displacement from superior osteotomy edge and prosthesis-neck. (*E*) Confirmation of superior, posterior, and medial position of the left prosthetic condylar head relative to the prosthetic fossa.

- Recommend avoidance of heavy-elastics and/or rigid MMF given risk of maxillary displacement.

Immediate postoperative care

- Recommend compression wrap around entire face
- Recommend near-constant ice therapy for the first 3 days
- Consider guiding orthodontic elastics to assist mandibular opening and closing, with maintenance of occlusion
  - Masticatory muscles are stripped from mandible so mandibular hypomobility and/or fatigue are expected
- When Le Fort I osteotomy was performed: recommend no-chew blenderized diet for at least 6 weeks
  - Patient will advance to regular-compromised diet and initiate postoperative orthodontics thereafter.
- Recommend initiation of gentle mandibular physical therapy within 1 week, with avoidance of joint-loading exercises until 6 weeks postoperatively.

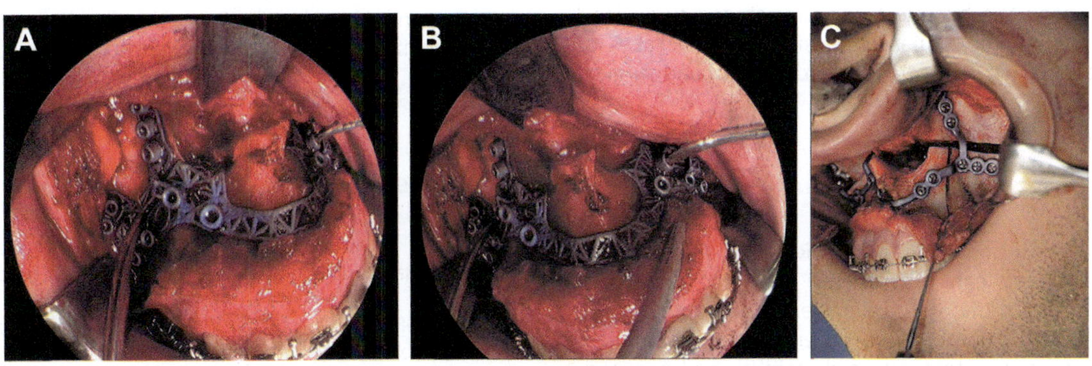

Fig. 16 (*A*) Confirmation of adaptation of single-piece maxillary cutting guide, with titanium tabs hooking onto the inferior piriform rim on the right. (*B*) Confirmation of adaptation of single-piece maxillary cutting guide, with titanium tabs hooking onto the inferior piriform rims bilaterally. (*C*) Extraoral view of fixated patient-specific hardware after guided-osteotomies.

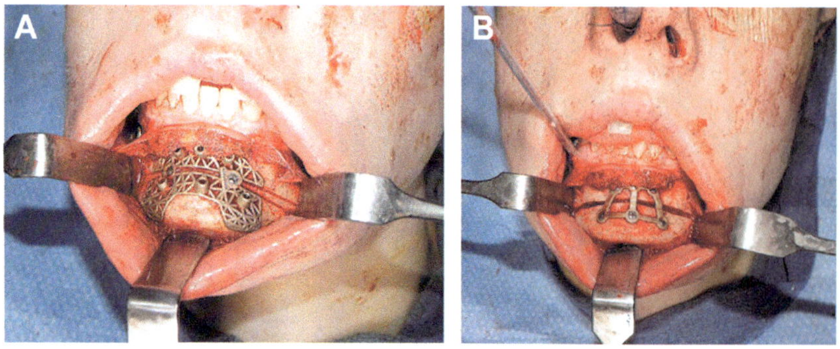

Fig. 17 (*A*) Extra-oral view of patient-specific genioplasty cutting guide. (*B*) Extra-oral view of fixated patient-specific genioplasty hardware.

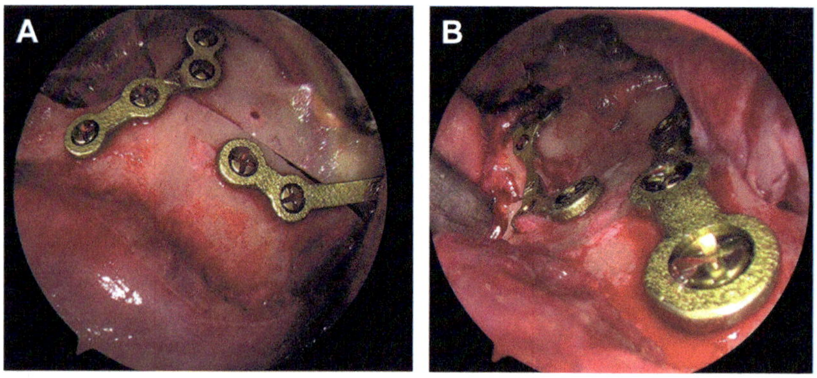

Fig. 18 (*A*) Appropriate adaptation of patient-specific left maxillary fixation plates, with the patient in intermaxillary fixation. (*B*) Appropriate adaptation of patient-specific right maxillary fixation plates, with the patient in intermaxillary fixation.

Rehabilitation and recovery

- Individualized postoperative physiotherapy is recommended, with more aggressive regimens used in patients with a history of preoperative mandibular hypomobility.
- Recommend utilization of formal, in-person physical therapy for soft tissue mobilization (reduction in edema), postural training, neuromuscular retraining, facial animation exercises, and improvement in mandibular range of motion.

Clinical results in the literature

- Limited studies have evaluated outcomes following combined TJR and orthognathics, as recent advancements have obviated the historical need for staged surgeries.[3] Preliminary studies demonstrate similarly low rates of complications with attention toward sterility and surgical technique.[4,5]

Summary

Pursuit and execution of TMJ TJR and simultaneous orthognathic surgery can provide life changing functional and esthetic improvements for patients presenting with end-stage TMJ arthropathies and dentofacial anomalies. Judicious planning is necessary; predictability and accuracy may be further supplemented with utilization of patient-specific osteotomy (cutting) guides, fixation guides, and PSI(s).

Clinics care points

- Pearls of combined TMJ-orthognathic reconstruction include: Diligent pre-operative planning, ensuring accurate models are used for planning of patient-specific hardware. Consideration of sequencing and diligence towards sterility are paramount to decrease highest risk (prosthetic joint infection).[7]
- Pitfalls of combined TMJ-orthognathic reconstruction include: Failure to achieve occlusion and/or correct position of positioning-guides and surgical guides; Failure to recognize malposition of TMJ prosthetic components and/or orthognathic hardware; failure to recognize development of dental malocclusion after plating.

References

1. Burris BJ, Bavarian R, Shaefer JR. Nonsurgical management of temporomandibular joint arthropathy. Dent Clin North Am 2023;67(1):27–47. PMID: 36404079.
2. Bouloux GF, Chou J, DiFabio V, et al. The contemporary management of temporomandibular joint intra-articular pain and dysfunction. J Oral Maxillofac Surg 2024;82(6):623–31. Epub 2024 Jan 6. PMID: 38280727.
3. Sembronio S, Robiony T, Robiony M. Protocol for fully digital and customized management of concomitant temporomandibular joint

replacement and orthognathic surgery. Int J Oral Maxillofac Surg 2021;50(2):212–9. ISSN 0901-5027.
4. Wolford LM, Mercuri LG. Concomitant TMJ total joint replacement and orthognathic surgery. In: Wolford L, editor. Temporomandibular joint total joint replacement – TMJ TJR. London, UK: Springer International Publishing; 2016. p. 133–63.
5. Amarista F, Perez D. Concomitant temporomandibular joint replacement and orthognathic surgery. Diagnostics (Basel) 2023;13(15):2486.
6. Daifallah TA, Margolis D, Haggerty CJ, et al. Concomitant temporomandibular joint replacement and orthognathic surgery. In: Haggerty CJ, Laughlin RM, editors. Atlas of operative oral and maxillofacial surgery. Hoboken (NJ): John Wiley & Sons, Inc; 2022. p. 619–36.
7. Warburton G, Mercuri LG. Alloplastic reconstruction of the temporomandibular joint in patients with dentofacial deformities. Atlas Oral Maxillofac Surg Clin North Am 2022;30(2):223–33.

Complications, Revision Surgery, and Rehabilitation

David Ahn, DMD [a], Jonathan Bensing, DMD, ML [b,*], Jordan Cimilluca, DDS [c], Hannah Jeffress-Vanders, DDS [c], Rebeka Silva, DMD, FACD [d]

KEYWORDS

• Temporomandibular joint • Total joint replacement • Complications • Revision surgery • Heterotopic ossification • Synovial entrapment • Alloplastic prosthesis

KEY POINTS

- Complications of temporomandibular joint (TMJ) total joint replacement include facial nerve injury, infection, heterotopic ossification, hardware failure, and synovial entrapment, requiring prompt management.
- Revision TMJ surgery demands meticulous preoperative evaluation, including detailed surgical history, high-resolution computed tomography imaging, and consideration of staged reconstruction in complex cases.
- Structured postoperative physiotherapy significantly improves range of motion, pain, and masticatory function and is essential to prevent reankylosis following open TMJ surgery.

Introduction

Complications following temporomandibular joint (TMJ) surgery are diverse and present unique challenges for the TMJ surgeon. Risk of complications increases in proportion to surgical complexity, as well as with prior interventions, anatomic alterations, and patient comorbidities. Effective management of TMJ surgical complications requires not only prompt recognition and comprehensive understanding of their etiology and strategies for prevention. This article provides an overview of various complications related to open joint procedures with a particular focus on total alloplastic TMJ replacement surgery.

Neurologic complications: facial nerve injury

Facial nerve injury, although rarely permanent, remains a commonly reported complication of TMJ total joint replacement (TJR) (Figs. 1–3). A systematic review by Peres Lima and colleagues reported facial nerve paresis or paralysis as the most prevalent complication of total joint replacement, occurring in 7.8% of cases.[1] The vast majority of deficits are transient, with normal function returning within 9 to 14 weeks, though permanent injury has been documented in rare cases.[2] Identification of key tissue planes remains paramount during dissection to the TMJ, including ensuring that anterior dissection along the lateral aspect of the zygomatic arch is performed in a subperiosteal plane, deep to the temporal branch of the facial nerve. The surgical team should also avoid excessive inferior retraction within a preauricular incision to minimize traction injury to the trunk of the facial nerve.

Periprosthetic joint infection

A retrospective survey of 2,476 TJR cases involving 3,368 joints, Mercuri reported a surgical site infection rate of 1.51%,[3] similar to the incidence of 2.5% of patients or 1.6% of all prostheses reported by Wolford.[4] Acute infections, defined by Wolford as those diagnosed and treated within 2 to 5 days of symptom onset, may be effectively managed with irrigation, debridement, and targeted antibiotic therapy, with reported prosthesis salvage rates approaching 80%. In contrast, chronic infections require a staged approach involving prosthesis removal, placement of an antibiotic spacer, and delayed reimplantation.[4] Prevention strategies include meticulous preoperative risk assessment, appropriately timed antibiotic prophylaxis, strict adherence to sterile technique, careful intraoperative hemostasis and tissue handling, and vigilant postoperative surveillance.[3]

Hardware failure

Hardware failure in TMJ TJR may present as screw loosening, fracture of fixation screws or prosthetic components (fossa or mandibular), and prosthesis displacement (see Figs. 2 and 3). Ettinger and colleagues demonstrated that increasing the number of fixation screws in the condylar component reduces

[a] Department of Oral and Maxillofacial Surgery, University of California, San Francisco VA Medical Center, 4150 Clement Street, San Francisco, CA 94121, USA
[b] Department of Oral & Maxillofacial Surgery, Walter Reed National Military Medical Center, 4494 Palmer Road N, Bethesda, MD 20814, USA
[c] Department of Oral and Maxillofacial Surgery, Uniformed Services University, Walter Reed National Military Medical Center, 4494 Palmer Roadd N, Bethesda, MD 20814, USA
[d] Division of Dental Service, Department of Oral & Maxillofacial Surgery, San Francisco VA Medical Center, 4150 Clement Street, San Francisco, CA 94121, USA
* Corresponding author.
E-mail address: jonathan.r.bening.mil@health.mil

1061-3315/26/
https://doi.org/10.1016/j.cxom.2026.05.008
oralmaxsurgeryatlas.theclinics.com

Abbreviations

CT computed tomography
HO heterotopic ossification
IMA internal maxillary artery
TJR total joint replacement
TMJ temporomandibular joint

per-screw stress and may decrease the risk of hardware failure.[5] Although relatively uncommon with contemporary prosthetic systems, hardware failure was more prevalent in historical designs, including the Christensen TMJ prosthesis, in which fossa component fractures were frequently observed during revision.[6] Trauma represents an additional mechanism of failure; fractures of mandibular ramus screws with associated prosthesis displacement have been reported following falls and other blunt force injuries, often necessitating device replacement. Hardware failure is typically treated with removal and replacement of the prosthesis. Strategic placement of new screws to avoid previously occupied or compromised bone can optimize fixation and reduce the risk of repeat failure.

Implant exposure and dehiscence

Implant exposure may occur through a preauricular incision, submandibular incision, or intraorally along the mandibular ramus (Fig. 4). Contributing factors include thin soft tissue coverage, previous irradiation (as in cases of osteoradionecrosis requiring reconstruction), poor wound healing, and chronic low-grade infection. Management typically requires soft tissue debridement, local or regional flap coverage, and in refractory cases, prosthesis removal with staged reconstruction. In complex cases involving prior radiation, microvascular free tissue transfer such as fibular free flap may be required for definitive reconstruction.

Heterotopic ossification

Heterotopic ossification (HO) is one of the most frequently cited reasons for TJR revision surgery (Fig. 5), reported as high as 20% in the absence of prophylactic measures.[7] HO can result in progressive limitation of mouth opening, reankylosis, and the need for revision surgery. The etiology is multifactorial and may involve periosteal disruption, residual bone fragments, and the patient's inherent osteogenic potential.

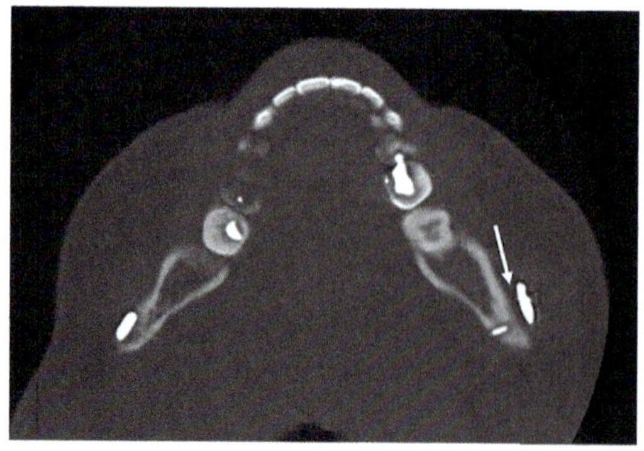

Fig. 2 Computed tomography (CT) imaging of a left TMJ prosthesis with screw fracture and prosthesis displacement. Note the gap between the lateral mandibular cortex and prosthesis (*arrow*).

Autologous fat grafting has emerged as the primary prophylactic measure against HO formation (Figs. 6 and 7). Wolford and Karras published the first study of this technique for TMJ TJR in 1997 and subsequent investigations have demonstrated a substantial reduction in HO rates to less than 5% when autologous fat is packed around the articulating components of the prosthesis.[8] In patients who develop recurrent HO despite fat grafting, management typically involves atraumatic prosthesis removal, thorough resection of heterotopic bone, replacement of the prosthesis, and reapplication of autologous fat around the articulation.

Intraoperative bleeding

Preoperative internal maxillary artery (IMA) embolization is a well-established adjunct for decreasing blood loss during open TMJ procedures, especially in cases of ankylosis release and TJR. A recent 10-year institutional experience of 73 patients (108 sides) undergoing preoperative IMA embolization before TMJ replacement demonstrated median operative blood loss of only 100 mL per side (interquartile range [IQR] 50–181 mL), with half the number of patients experiencing excessive blood loss compared to historical controls (12.5% vs 25%).[9] The procedure is typically performed using coils (Fig. 8) with a median of 3 coils per side, sometimes combined with n-butyl cyanoacrylate (glue); the middle meningeal artery may also be occluded in approximately 26% of cases.[10]

Embolization is generally performed 24 to 48 hours before surgery and surgery should proceed within this window to prevent collateral revascularization. Preoperative CT angiography is essential to assess the relationship between the

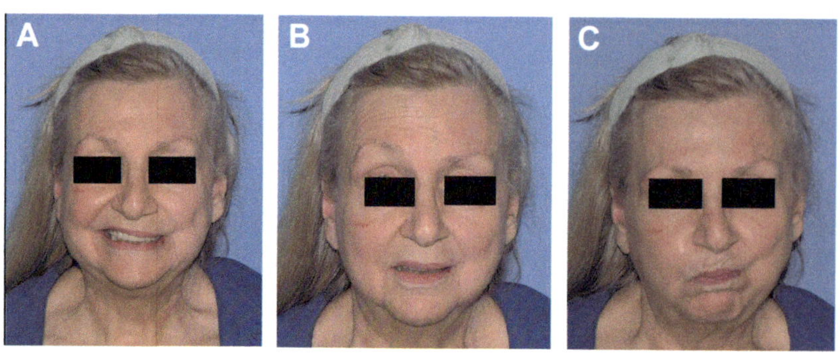

Fig. 1 (*A–C*) A patient with history of multiple TMJ surgeries resulting in damage to the facial nerve.

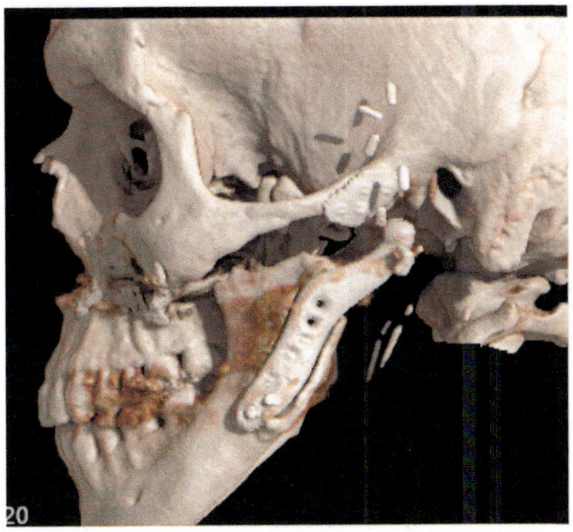

Fig. 3 CT imaging 3D reconstruction of patient with screw failure and displacement of mandibular prosthesis.

IMA/external carotid artery and the ankylotic mass or surgical field, with embolization indicated when intimate anatomic association is present.

Synovial entrapment

Identifying the cause of periprosthetic pain and limited mandibular opening after TMJ TJR can be challenging, with a broad differential that includes myofascial pain, centrally mediated pain, and other postoperative complications. When clinical and radiographic findings do not reveal a clear etiology, synovial entrapment should be considered. Also referred to as synovial impingement, synovial entrapment occurs when synovial tissue proliferates and becomes interposed within the articulating surfaces of prosthesis. This phenomenon has been described in hip and knee arthroplasty as well as in both stock and patient-specific TMJ prostheses.[11] Synovial entrapment is rarely reported, likely because definitive diagnosis typically requires surgical exploration of the prosthetic joint since soft tissue ingrowth may not be visualized on radiographic workup. Management generally involves open or arthroscopic debridement of soft tissue interposed between the prosthetic components.[12] Histopathologic evaluation of the periprosthetic

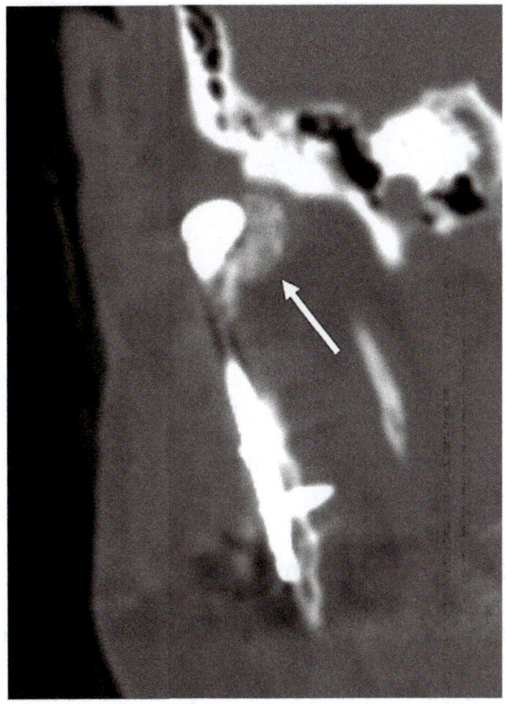

Fig. 5 Periprosthetic heterotopic ossification (*arrow*) medial to the condylar component.

pseudocapsular tissue can confirm the presence or absence of entrapped synovium.

Figs. 9 and 10 show the left total joint replacement of a 65 year old female 5 years after placement of the prosthesis. In the years before her revision surgery, the patient began to experience progressive joint pain with function and decreased oral opening. Without other significant findings on clinical examination and CT imaging negative for signs of prosthetic failure, the patient was taken to the operating room for open exploration of the prosthesis. Upon access to the joint, a soft tissue encapsulation of the condylar component was identified, occupying the space between the articulating surfaces (see Fig. 9 arrow). This tissue was removed with hand instrumentation (see Fig. 10) and sent for histopathologic analysis. Biopsy results confirmed reactive synovium with degenerative changes.

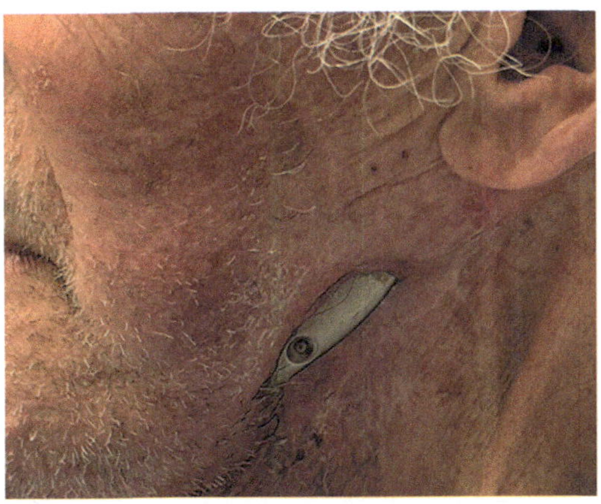

Fig. 4 Left TMJ TJR implant exposure in a patient with a history of head and neck radiation.

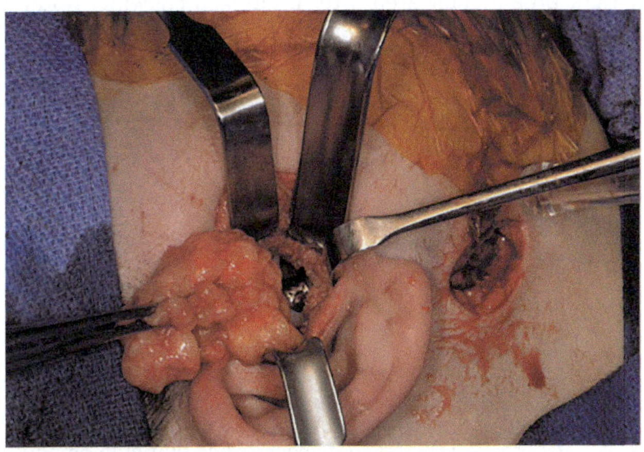

Fig. 6 Autologous fat graft positioned over TJR surgical site. The prosthesis is visible within the incision.

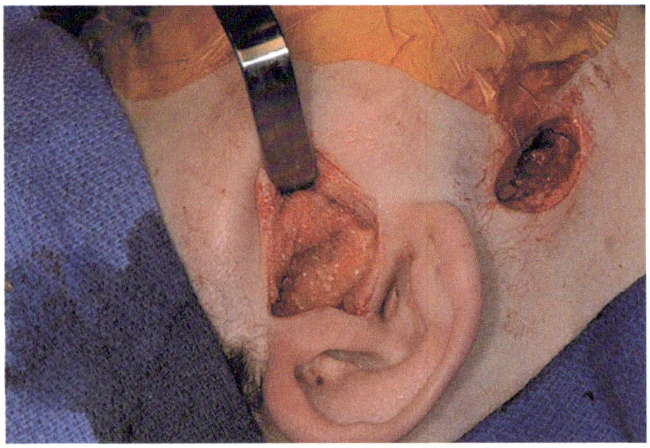

Fig. 7 Fat graft has been packed into the surgical site around the prosthesis.

Poor prosthesis biocompatibility

Before the development of modern TMJ prostheses, much controversy was generated by TMJ implants later found to be the source of significant long-term complications. Most notably, Proplast–Teflon implants—interpositional devices composed of a porous Proplast surface intended for apposition to the temporal bone and a Teflon (PTFE) surface articulating with the mandibular condyle—were widely used throughout the 1970s and 1980s. While this prosthesis gained early acceptance, reports of delayed, but severe foreign body giant cell reactions and particle-induced osteolysis led to their eventual abandonment and recall.[13,14] Over time, implant fragmentation was frequently observed, resulting in robust inflammatory responses and progressive destruction of both the mandibular condyle and glenoid fossa. In advanced cases, osteolysis has been reported to extend superiorly toward the cranial base and middle cranial fossa, creating substantial reconstructive challenges and increasing the risk of intracranial complications.[14,15]

Revision total joint replacement surgery

A 75-year-old female with a history of multiple prior TMJ surgeries, including placement of bilateral TMJ Proplast-Teflon implants, presents with complaint of right TMJ pain. The patient endorses right TMJ clicking, decreased opening, and swelling of her right preauricular area after prolonged chewing. Notably, she reports concern that her mandible has drifted posteriorly.

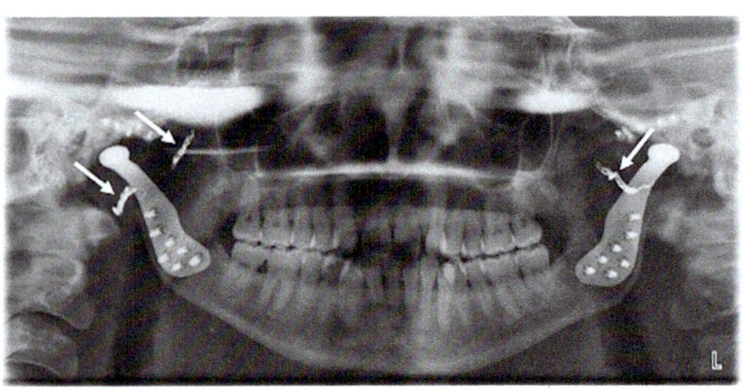

Fig. 8 Panoramic radiograph demonstrating platinum embolization coils (*arrows*) placed during embolization of bilateral internal maxillary arteries.

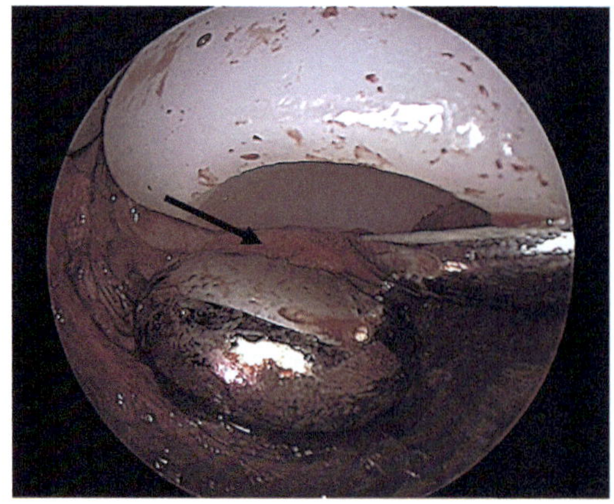

Fig. 9 Soft tissue ingrowth (*arrow*) into TMJ TJR articulating surfaces.

Preoperative evaluation and planning

Preoperative evaluation of this patient, as always, begins with a thorough patient history including detailed review of any past TMJ procedures, followed by physical examination with careful documentation of baseline facial nerve function, TMJ function, and occlusion. CT imaging with thin cuts and 3-dimensional reconstruction is essential in revision TMJ surgery. In this patient, CT imaging is notable for erosion of the right glenoid fossa with perforation into the middle cranial fossa (Figs. 11 and 12). When soft tissue pathology or intracranial extension is suspected based on clinical examination or CT imaging, MRI may provide additional information regarding synovial proliferation, joint effusion, or potential dural involvement.

In cases such as this with involvement of the middle cranial fossa involvement, coordination with neurosurgical colleagues should be considered, particularly if there is concern for dural exposure or intracranial involvement during implant removal. In revision TJR surgery, single-stage reconstruction versus staged surgical approaches must be considered. In cases involving infection, severe inflammatory reaction, extensive osteolysis, or significant bone loss, a staged approach is often preferred. The initial procedure focuses on removal of the failed implant material and thorough debridement of inflammatory or reactive tissue. Placement of an antibiotic-impregnated polymethyl methacrylate spacer may be used to

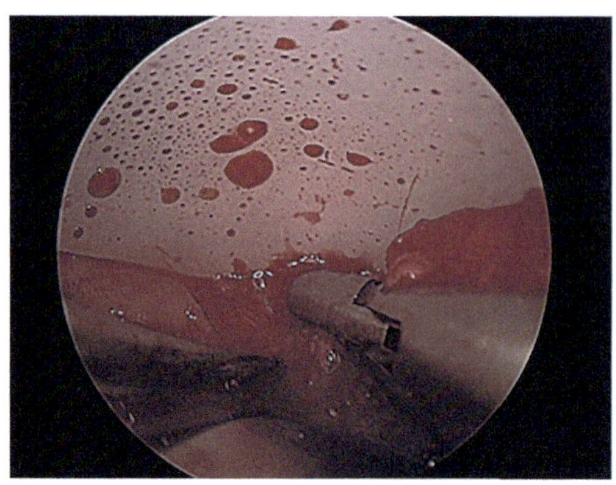

Fig. 10 Surgical debridement of soft tissue impingement visualized.

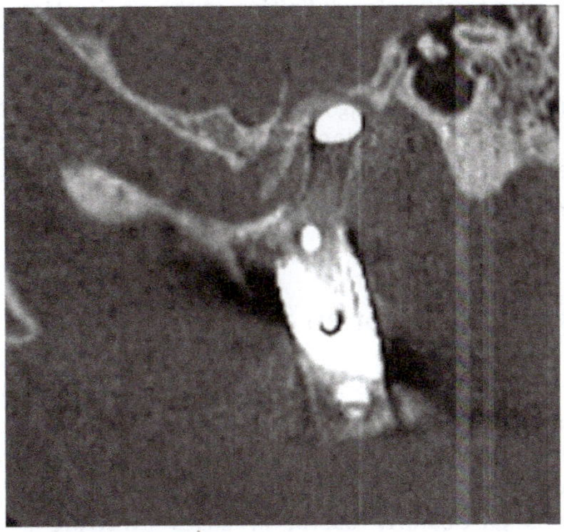

Fig. 11 Sagittal CT image demonstrating erosion of the right glenoid fossa with superior extension and perforation into the middle cranial fossa.

maintain joint space and allow soft tissue recovery before definitive reconstruction.[16,17]

In this case, a custom TMJ TJR is selected for definitive reconstruction. Given the altered bony anatomy of the right cranial base, a patient-specific fossa allows strategically placed fixation and protection of the middle cranial fossa perforation. Selection of a custom prosthesis also supports a 2-staged reconstruction as removing existing hardware will avoid metal artifacts on imaging that would otherwise make virtual surgical planning and prosthesis manufacturing difficult.

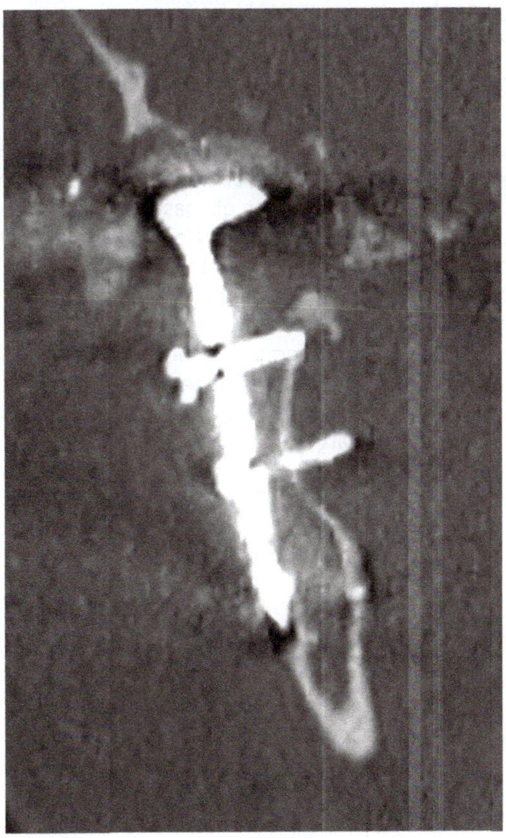

Fig. 12 Coronal CT image confirming right glenoid fossa erosion with intracranial extension into the middle cranial fossa.

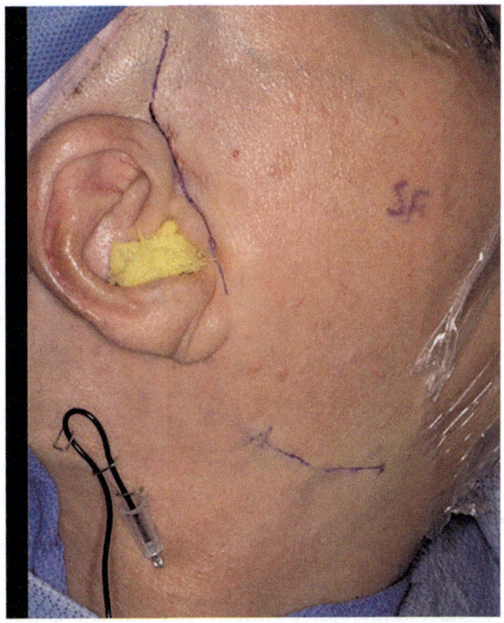

Fig. 13 Example of marked preauricular and submandibular incisions, as well as a nerve monitor electrode placed in the sternocleidomastoid muscle.

Step 1 surgical access to the temporomandibular joint and removal of the failed prosthesis

This procedure is performed under general anesthesia with nasotracheal intubation to allow intraoperative assessment of

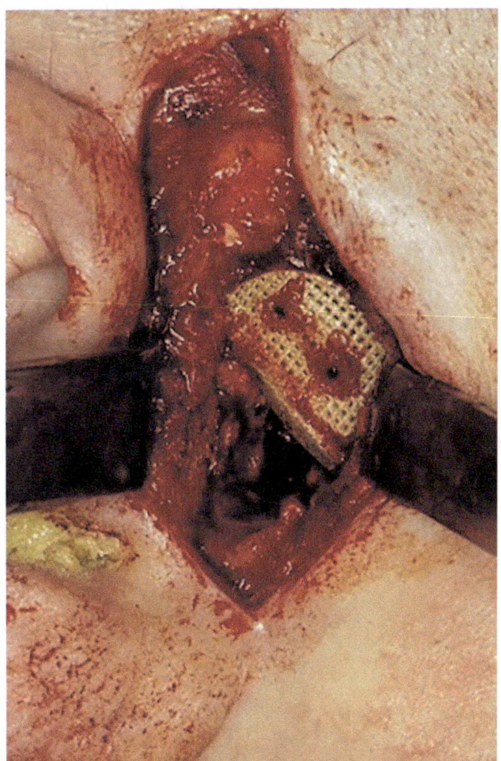

Fig. 14 Intraoperative photograph showing exposure through a preauricular approach with identification and removal of the Proplast–Teflon implant from the posterior zygomatic arch region.

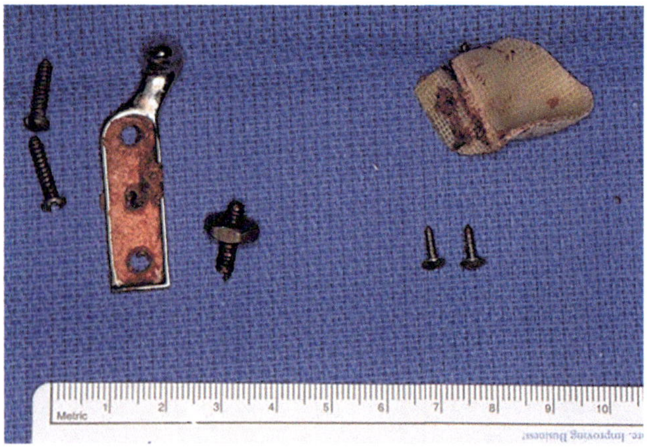

Fig. 15 Explanted Proplast–Teflon implant and associated fixation hardware following removal, including screws and plate components.

occlusion and mandibular position. The patient is positioned supine with the head rotated contralaterally to expose the operative side. The temporal, preauricular, and mandibular regions were prepared and draped in a sterile fashion. Revision TMJ surgery typically uses a combined preauricular or endaural approach with a submandibular or retromandibular approach to allow adequate access to both the glenoid fossa and the mandibular ramus (Fig. 13).

To ensure protection of the facial nerve, intraoperative facial nerve monitoring is used to guide dissection in a surgical field where scar tissue obscured normal anatomic landmarks. Nerve monitoring systems such as the Nerve Integrity Monitoring System or handheld stimulators such as the Checkpoint nerve stimulator can be used for this purpose (see Fig. 13).

Dissection from the preauricular incision was continued through the scarred tissue planes to the posterior zygomatic arch where the existing Proplast-Teflon implant was identified. The implant and all fixation hardware were removed (Figs. 14 and 15). Debridement of inflammatory or fibrotic tissue is essential to eliminate reactive tissue and improve the local biological environment for reconstruction.

Step 2 management of cranial base defect

The cranial base deep to the Proplast-Teflon implant is carefully evaluated given the radiographic evidence of erosion into the middle cranial fossa. Granulomatous tissue was removed from the area to allow for definition of the perforation margins and dural integrity. In such cases, small bony defects may be managed with autogenous grafts, alloplastic materials, or soft tissue coverage, depending on the extent of the defect and the overall reconstructive plan. In this case, a neurosurgery consultation is obtained for evaluation of the defect intraoperatively, which is temporarily covered with a collagen-derived matrix (Fig. 16).

Step 3 placement of an antibiotic spacer

Following removal of the failed prosthesis and completion of debridement, placement of an antibiotic-impregnated polymethyl methacrylate spacer is performed to maintain the joint space and surrounding soft tissue envelope (Fig. 17). This strategy is particularly useful in cases involving infection, extensive inflammatory reaction, or severe bone loss.

Step 4 staged reconstruction with total joint prosthesis

After resolution of inflammation and adequate healing of the surgical site, a second-stage procedure is performed for definitive TMJ reconstruction using a custom total joint prosthesis. The joint is reexposed through the previous surgical approaches and the antibiotic spacer is removed. A custom TMJ prosthesis is then placed with the fossa component designed to protect the area of bony erosion and to allow for adequate fixation despite altered anatomy. Proper positioning of the prosthesis is ensured to restore vertical ramus height, establish stable occlusion, and maintain appropriate mandibular alignment.

Postoperative physiotherapy and rehabilitation

Regardless of the specific surgical intervention, rehabilitation goals should include restoration of functional range of motion, reduction of pain, improvement of masticatory function, and prevention of postsurgical complications such as reankylosis. De Meurechy and colleagues conducted a systematic review of physiotherapy after open TMJ surgery and proposed a 3-step rehabilitation program: (1) an early postoperative phase (weeks 1–2) focusing on edema control, gentle passive range-of-motion exercises, and pain management; (2) an intermediate phase (weeks 3–6) introducing progressive active-assisted and active exercises targeting mouth opening, lateral excursions, and protrusion; and (3) a late phase (weeks 7–12 and

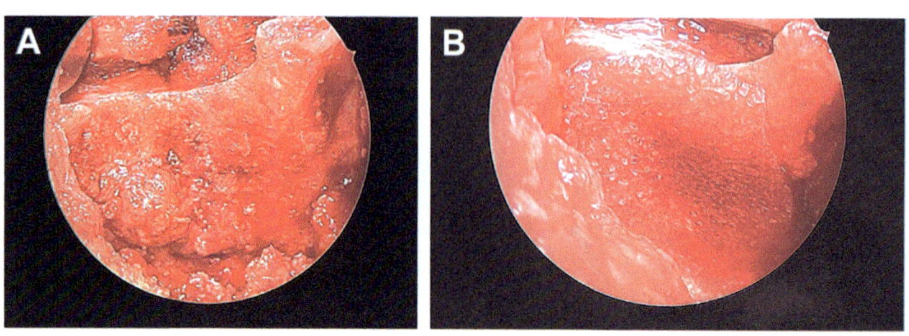

Fig. 16 (*A, B*) Endoscopic view of the glenoid fossa defect with dural exposure. Collagen matrix placed for temporary coverage of the defect.

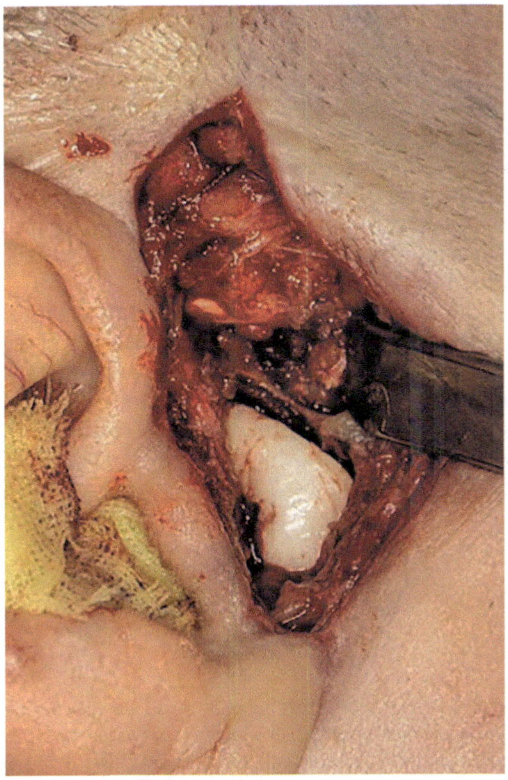

Fig. 17 Placement of antibiotic spacer.

beyond) emphasizing strengthening, functional retraining, and parafunctional habit modification. Overall, patients in the reviewed studies demonstrated significant improvements in range of motion (+9.8 mm), pain scores (−5.2 points on visual analog scale), and diet and chewing scores (+1.7 points).[18] One adjunct device includes the TheraBite Jaw Motion Rehab System (Fig. 18), a handheld device that allows patients to set their goal maximum opening.

Pearls and pitfalls

- *Ensure a comprehensive workup is complete prior to planning revision surgery*

Although it may be tempting to expedite revision surgery in an effort to *correct* prior procedures, a thorough, detailed workup is essential. Careful review of the patient's history, repeat imaging, and appropriate serologic studies are critical components that contribute to optimal surgical outcomes.

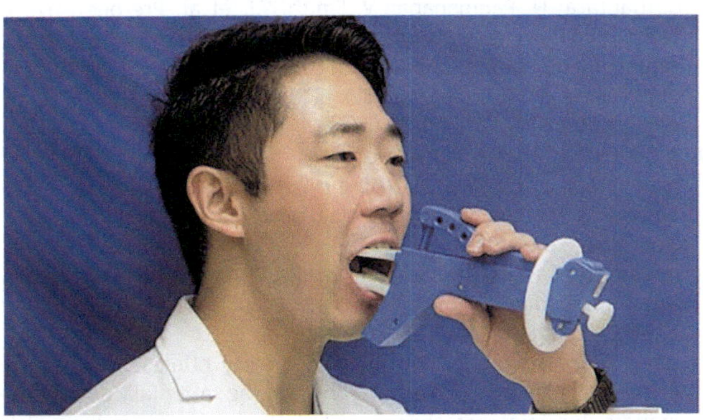

Fig. 18 Example of TheraBite in use. TheraBite Jaw Motion Rehabilitation System. Used with permission from Atos Medical.

- *Rule out nonsurgical etiologies of patient symptoms*

Similar to treatment-naïve patients, those with previous TMJ surgery may experience symptoms of myofascial pain, centralized pain, muscular dystonia, and manifestations of psychiatric disorders. These etiologies may be more appropriately managed with nonsurgical therapies and should be carefully considered before revision surgical intervention.

- *Minimize risk of prosthesis dislocation through careful surgical planning and technique*

Improper positioning of the fossa and mandibular components increases the risk of prosthetic instability and dislocation. Intraoperatively, adequate resection at the condylectomy site must be confirmed to prevent bony interferences that may lateralize the condylar component (Fig. 19). The fossa component should be fully seated before fixation; application of superior-medial pressure during fixation facilitates accurate positioning. As illustrated in Fig. 20, improper seating may result in a gap between the patient-specific fossa and the temporal bone. Postoperative otalgia may result from a posteriorly malpositioned fossa.[19]

- *Establish realistic expectations for both surgeon and patient*

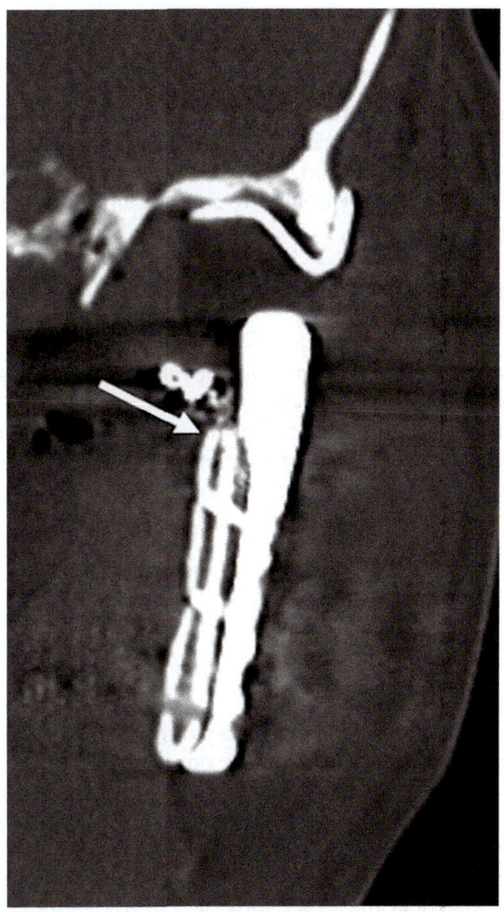

Fig. 19 Postoperative CT scan showing inadequate reduction during the condylectomy (*arrow*), with bony interference causing lateralization of the mandibular component.

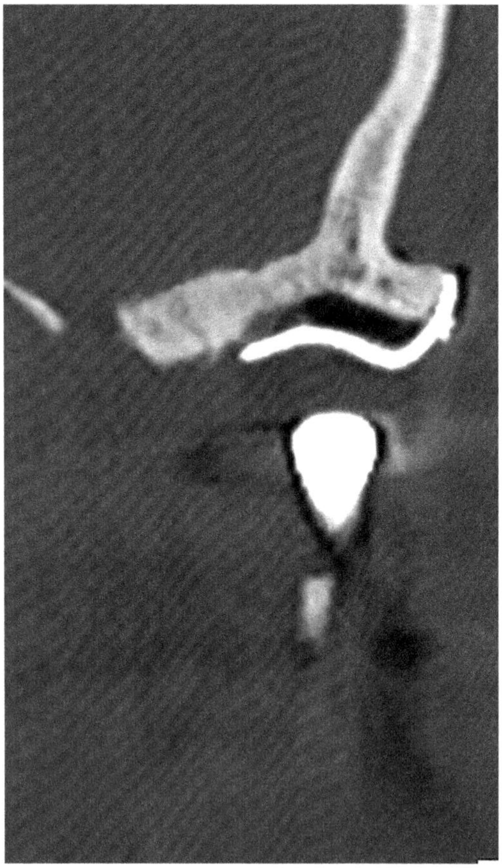

Fig. 20 Postoperative CT scan demonstrating a gap between the prosthetic fossa and native bony fossa.

The degree of symptom improvement following revision TMJ surgery may be less pronounced than that achieved with primary surgical intervention.[20] Clear communication regarding expected outcomes is essential to support appropriate patient management.

- *Emphasize postoperative physiotherapy to maintain results*

Perioperative care extends well beyond the operating room. Early mobilization and structured physiotherapy are essential to minimize scar formation and prevent loss of range of motion following revision surgery. Surgeons should proactively educate patients on the importance of rehabilitation protocols.

Clinics care points

- Successful revision surgery depends not only on prosthesis replacement but also on identifying and correcting the underlying cause of failure, including infection, heterotopic ossification, implant malposition, or soft tissue impingement.
- Facial nerve injury risk is increased during revision and multiply operated TMJ surgery. Careful preoperative documentation of facial nerve function establishes a baseline for postoperative assessment, while meticulous soft tissue handling and avoidance of excessive retraction help minimize nerve injury.
- Acute periprosthetic infection may be successfully managed with irrigation, debridement, and targeted antibiotics, whereas chronic infection generally requires prosthesis removal and staged reconstruction.
- Autologous fat grafting around the articulating components remains the most effective strategy for preventing heterotopic ossification following TMJ total joint replacement.
- Preoperative internal maxillary artery embolization should be considered for complex ankylosis and revision cases to reduce intraoperative blood loss.
- Progressive pain and restricted mandibular opening despite normal imaging should raise suspicion for synovial entrapment, which often requires surgical exploration for diagnosis.

References

1. Peres Lima FGG, Rios LGC, Bianchi J, et al. Complications of total temporomandibular joint replacement: a systematic review and meta-analysis. Int J Oral Maxillofac Surg 2023;52(5):584–94.
2. Moin A, Shetty AD, Archana TS, et al. Facial nerve injury in temporomandibular joint approaches. Ann Maxillofac Surg 2018;8(1):51–5.
3. Mercuri LG. Avoiding and managing temporomandibular joint total joint replacement surgical site infections. J Oral Maxillofac Surg 2012;70(10):2280–9.
4. Wolford LM, Rodrigues DB, McPhillips A. Management of the infected temporomandibular joint total joint prosthesis. J Oral Maxillofac Surg 2010;68(11):2810–23.
5. Ettinger KS, Arce K, Fillmore WJ, et al. Does the amount of screw fixation utilized for the condylar component of the TMJ concepts total temporomandibular joint reconstruction predispose to hardware loss or postoperative complications? J Oral Maxillofac Surg 2016;74(9):1741–50.
6. Wolford LM. Factors to consider in joint prosthesis systems. Proc (Bayl Univ Med Cent) 2006;19(3):232.
7. Almeida LE, Zammuto S, Mercuri LG. Quality of life outcomes following total temporomandibular joint replacement: a systematic review of long-term efficacy, functional improvements, and complication rates across prosthesis types. J Clin Med 2025;14(14). https://doi.org/10.3390/JCM14144859.
8. Mercuri LG, Ali FA, Woolson R. Outcomes of total alloplastic replacement with periarticular autogenous fat grafting for management of reankylosis of the temporomandibular joint. J Oral Maxillofac Surg 2008;66(9):1794–803.
9. Sujijantarat N, Padmanaban V, Smith WJ, et al. Pre-operative internal maxillary artery embolization for temporomandibular joint replacement: safety and outcomes from a 10-year institutional experience. J Neurointerventional Surg 2026;18(2). https://doi.org/10.1136/JNIS-2024-022975.
10. Alderazi YJ, Shastri D, Wessel J, et al. Internal maxillary artery preoperative embolization using n-Butyl cyanoacrylate and pushable coils for temporomandibular joint ankylosis surgery. World Neurosurg 2017;101:254–8.
11. Ângelo DF, Cardoso HJ, Sanz D. Synovial entrapment in alloplastic temporomandibular joint replacement. Int J Oral Maxillofac Surg 2021;50(12):1628–31.
12. Davis CM, Hakim M, Choi DD, et al. Early clinical outcomes of arthroscopic management of the failing alloplastic temporomandibular joint prosthesis. J Oral Maxillofac Surg 2020;78(6):903–7.

13. Lee KC, Eisig SB, Perrino MA. Foreign body giant cell reaction to a proplast/teflon interpositional implant: a case report and literature review. J Oral Maxillofac Surg 2018;76(8):1719–24.
14. Schellhas KP, Wilkes CH, El Deeb M, et al. Permanent proplast temporomandibular joint implants: MR imaging of destructive complications. AJR Am J Roentgenol 1988;151(4):731–5.
15. Sahdev R, Wu BW, Anderson N, et al. A retrospective study of patient outcomes after temporomandibular joint replacement with alloplastic total joint prosthesis at Massachusetts general hospital. J Oral Maxillofac Surg 2019;77(2):280–8.
16. Zaid WY, Alshehry S, Zakhary G, et al. Use of vascularized myo-osseous fibula free flap to reconstruct a hemimandibular defect with a concomitant skull defect arising from stock condylar prosthesis displacement into the middle cranial fossa. J Oral Maxillofac Surg 2019;77(6):1316.e1–12.
17. Teschke M, Christensen A, Far F, et al. Digitally designed, personalized bone cement spacer for staged TMJ and mandibular reconstruction - introduction of a new technique. J Craniomaxillofac Surg 2021;49(10):935–42.
18. De Meurechy NKG, Loos PJ, Mommaerts MY. Postoperative physiotherapy after open temporomandibular joint surgery: a 3-Step program. J Oral Maxillofac Surg 2019;77(5):932–50.
19. Ghaly GA, Espeso A, McIntyre G. Temporomandibular joint alloplastic replacement failure. Br J Oral Maxillofac Surg 2024;62(9):848–56.
20. Gakhal MK, Gupta B, Sidebottom AJ. Analysis of outcomes after revision replacement of failed total temporomandibular joint prostheses. Br J Oral Maxillofac Surg 2020;58(2):220–4.

9780443474705